Lecture Notes in Computer Science   10219

Commenced Publication in 1973
Founding and Former Series Editors:
Gerhard Goos, Juris Hartmanis, and Jan van Leeuwen

More information about this series at http://www.springer.com/series/7409

Chunxiao Xing · Yong Zhang
Ye Liang (Eds.)

Smart Health

International Conference, ICSH 2016
Haikou, China, December 24–25, 2016
Revised Selected Papers

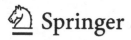 Springer

Editors
Chunxiao Xing
Tsinghua University
Beijing
China

Yong Zhang
Tsinghua University
Beijing
China

Ye Liang
Beijing Foreign Studies University
Beijing
China

ISSN 0302-9743   ISSN 1611-3349 (electronic)
Lecture Notes in Computer Science
ISBN 978-3-319-59857-4   ISBN 978-3-319-59858-1   (eBook)
DOI 10.1007/978-3-319-59858-1

Library of Congress Control Number: 2017941505

LNCS Sublibrary: SL3 – Information Systems and Applications, incl. Internet/Web, and HCI

Printed on acid-free paper

This Springer imprint is published by Springer Nature
The registered company is Springer International Publishing AG
The registered company address is: Gewerbestrasse 11, 6330 Cham, Switzerland

Preface

Advancing informatics for health care and health-care applications has become an international research priority. There is increased effort to transform reactive care to proactive and preventive care, clinic-centric to patient-centered practice, training-based interventions to globally aggregated evidence, and episodic response to continuous well-being monitoring and maintenance. The annual International Conference for Smart Health (ICSH) began in 2013. This first conference, held in Beijing, attracted over 50 contributors and participants from all over the world, providing a forum for meaningful multidisciplinary interactions.

The 2016 International Conference for Smart Health (ICSH 2016) was organized to develop a platform for authors to discuss fundamental principles, algorithms, or applications of intelligent data acquisition, processing, and analysis of health-care information. Specifically, this conference mainly focused on topics and issues including information sharing, integrating and extraction, clinical practice and medical monitoring, clinical and medical data mining, and large-scale health data analysis and management. We are pleased that many high-quality technical papers were submitted, accompanied by evaluation with real-world data or application contexts. The work presented at the conference encompassed a healthy mix of computer science, medical informatics, and information systems approaches.

ICSH 2016 was held in Haikou, China. The one-day event encompassed presentations of 23 papers. The organizers of ICSH 2016 would like to thank the conference sponsors for their support and sponsorship, including Hainan University, Tsinghua University, University of Arizona, Chinese Academy of Sciences, National Natural Science Foundation of China, and Beijing Biochem Hengye S&T Development Co., Ltd. We also greatly appreciate the following technical co-sponsors: Institute for Operations Research and the Management Sciences (INFORMS), ACM Beijing Chapter, and China Association for Information Systems. We further wish to express our sincere gratitude to all Program Committee members of ICSH 2016, who provided valuable and constructive review comments. This proceedings volume is supported by the Young Faculty Research Fund of Beijing Foreign Studies University under grant number 2015JT008. We further wish to express our sincere gratitude to all sponsors.

December 2016

Ye Liang
Chunxiao Xing
Hsinchun Chen

Organization

Conference Co-chairs

Hsinchun Chen   University of Arizona, USA
Daniel Zeng   University of Arizona, USA, and Chinese Academy
        of Sciences, China

Local Chair

Mengxing Huang   Hainan University, China

Workshop Co-chairs

Mengxing Huang   Hainan University, China
Ye Liang   Beijing Foreign Studies University, China

Publication Chair

Ye Liang   Beijing Foreign Studies University, China

Finance Chair

Yuanyuan Zhou   Tsinghua University, China

Publicity Chair

Yu Zhang   Hainan University, China

Local Arrangements Chair

Jingbin Li   Hainan University, China

Program Committee

Guanling Chen   University of Massachusetts Lowell, USA
Amar Das   Dartmouth College, USA
Ron Fricker   Naval Postgraduate School, USA
Natalia Grabar   STL CNRS Université Lille, France
Takahiro Hara   Osaka University, Japan
Xiaohua Hu   Drexel University, USA
Kun Huang   The Ohio State University, USA
Mengxing Huang   Hainan University, China

Roozbeh Jafari   University of Texas at Dallas, USA
Ernesto JimenezRuiz   University of Oxford, UK
Victor Jin   The Ohio State University, USA
Kenneth Komatsu   Arizona Department of Health Services, USA
Erhun Kundakcioglu   University of Houston, USA
Gondy Leroy   Claremont Graduate University, USA
Jiao Li   Chinese Academy of Medical Sciences, China
Ye Liang   Beijing Foreign Studies University, China
Mohammad Mahoor   University of Denver, USA
Radhakrishnan   University of Kentucky, USA
  Nagarajan
Xiaoming Sheng   University of Utah, USA
Min Song   New Jersey Institute of Technology, USA
Xing Tan   University of Ottawa, Canada
Chunqiang Tang   IBM T.J. Watson Research Center, USA
Cui Tao   Mayo Clinic, USA
Egon L. Van Den Broek   TNO/University of Twente/Radboud UMC Nijmegen,
                                The Netherlands
Jason Wang   New Jersey Institute of Technology, USA
May D. Wang   Georgia Institute of Technology and Emory University,
                                USA
Chunhua Weng   Columbia University, USA
Jinglong Wu   Okayama University, Japan
Bo Xie   University of Texas at Austin, USA
Chunxiao Xing   Tsinghua University, China
Hui Yang   University of South Florida, USA
Guigang Zhang   Chinese Academy of Sciences, China
Mi Zhang   University of Southern California, USA
Min Zhang   Peking University, China
Yong Zhang   Tsinghua University, China
Zhongming Zhao   Vanderbilt University, USA
Kai Zheng   The University of Michigan, USA

Contents

Medical Monitoring and Information Extraction, Clinical and Medical Data Mining

Big Data and Smart Health

The SWOT Analysis of the Wearable Devices in Smart Health Applications

Yu Yang[1], Sijun Yu[2(✉)], Yuwen Hao[1], Xiao Xu[3], and Huiliang Liu[2(✉)]

[1] Department of Medical Affairs, General Hospital of Chinese People's Armed Police Forces,
Beijing, China
yysbox@126.com, how_yuwen@163.com
[2] Department of Cardiology, General Hospital of Chinese People's Armed Police Forces,
Beijing, China
rdysj@163.com, lh1518@vip.sina.com
[3] Department of Dermatological Regeneration Medicine, General Hospital of Chinese People's
Armed Police Forces, Beijing, China
13623345@qq.com

Abstract. Proposed in recent years, smart health has gained great attention after its debut. Undoubtedly, wearable devices will bring great convenience to the development of smart health. With the aging trend, increase of empty families and solitary elderly people, and the growth spurt of chronic disease, wearable devices have come to its spring. But due to the lack of standards in the industry, the data collected by wearable devices is unreliable, and is difficult to be accepted by doctors. Besides, there are also some problems concerning with privacy. In this paper, the advantages, disadvantages, opportunities and obstacles of wearable devices are analyzed, and some development suggestions are provided.

Keywords: Smart health · Wearable device · SWOT

1 Introduction

According to data released by "Chinese chronic diseases prevention and control plan 2012–2015", which was issued by National Health and Family Planning Commission of the People's Republic of China in 2012, the number of China's chronic diseases patients is rising rapidly. The Confirmed Patients are over 260 million, and the deaths caused by chronic diseases account for 85% of the total number of deaths in China in 2012 [1]. Traditional ways of chronic diseases prevention and health management are far from enough demand, while the emergence of wearable devices has brought a glimmer of light for the development of medical field.

In August 2013, Premier Li Keqiang pointed out clearly at State Council meeting that encouraging commercial insurance companies to cooperate with wearable devices companies to foster customers through profit sharing model. This comment marks the bright future of wearable device development.

© Springer International Publishing AG 2017
C. Xing et al. (Eds.): ICSH 2016, LNCS 10219, pp. 3–8, 2017.
DOI: 10.1007/978-3-319-59858-1_1

2   The Concept of Wearable Medical Devices

2.1   The Concept of Wearable Medical Devices

Wearable device is a kind of portable device that can be weared directly, or integrated into the user's clothing or accessories. Wearable devices can be roughly classified as two categories: sports and health. This paper is mainly focused on the devices in the field of medical equipment. The wearable medical devices are some medical equipment that can be attached or wearing on people's body. And these equipments can be used in medical diagnosis, treatment and education training and scientific research, including real-time monitoring of patients' physiological process, transmitting data for analysis and review, and providing real-time communication and feedback between doctors and patients [2].

2.2   The Status Quo of Wearable Medical Devices

Since the concept of wearable device was put forward, some wearable products have sprung up. At present, there are dozens of wearable devices in the domestic market, such as intelligent thermometer, intelligent bracelet, intelligent blood oxygen meter, etc. The Dayima Company, which has more than tens of millions of active users, has successively introduced the intelligent thermometer and intelligent scales together with the Ruiren Company and PICOOC [3]. In October 2014, a kind of smart wearable equipment, named "upper arm type wireless electronic sphygmomanometer", which was invented independently by Guangzhou Huaqi digital company, was put on the market. And in 2015, Andon Health Co. Ltd. reached cooperation with Xiao mi Company, and launched the iHealth series products.

Wearable medical equipment started early in foreign countries, and the technologies is relatively mature. The MCOT (Mobile Cardiac Outpatient Telemetry) invented by American CardioNet Company, is able to not only record Patients electrocardiogram data within 30 days, but also to transmit the data to the monitoring center through the network. Then the analyzing and conclusion report will be sent to patients after the process. Once an abnormal heart rate of the patient is detected by the detector, it will be sent via the wireless terminal through the CDMA network to the monitoring center, where special medical personnel will record and analyze the data. Stanford University has invented a new wearable sensor. It is only a piece of paper thick and the same size as a stamp. Patients with heart disease may test heart rate anytime and anywhere by sticking it on his wrist [4].

There is a "dosing bra", designed for high-risk groups of breast cancer patients, which has TAMOXIFEN microcapsule bubble in its cover cup. In addition, Google is developing a contact lenses embedded a blood sugar level sensor measuring tears. While Apple is trying to perceive blood detection techniques applied to intelligent wearable devices. The Edison chip based on the Intel has also been applied to the design of Mimo baby clothes. Removable built-in sensors, fixed in a turtle shape clip, can get baby's physiological parameters in real-time, so that parents can monitor the child's physical condition at any time by the APP [5]. An intelligent tie for elder people also has Edison chip, the color of the tie will change while the wearer's mood changes. By this way, the tie may remind children to concern more about their parents' mental and fiscal health at any time.

3   The SWOT Analysis of the Wearable Medical Devices

3.1   Wearable Medical Devices' "Strength"

Real-time monitoring. Due to its nature of contacting with the human body for long time, wearable devices can collect data conveniently and timely. With the help of these devices, chronic diseases can be detected earlier by measuring the health indicators. Therefore, people can reduce the trouble of going to the hospital back and forth frequently. At the same time, the time cost and the economic cost of disease control are both reduced obviously. Comparatively speaking, under the traditional medical mode, it is difficult to accurately diagnose the patient due to the short contact time among doctors and patients. The purpose of early found, early treatment and early rehabilitation may be achieved through the whole testing, because the mode makes it easier to find the cause more rapid and more accurately.

Cost reduction. By connecting the wearable devices with the internet, the doctor can get the patient's physical condition over a long distance. The cost of both the patient and the doctor will be saved due to breaking the limitation by time and space. That most patients do not need to go to the hospital for examination, can not only reduce the patient's clinic time, but also reduce the congestion at hospital and the cost of the instruments and equipment space.

Medical big data. After the wearable devices become popular, the wearer's physiological data can be collected. Because of the large population base, the data collected if used properly afterwards, can play a key role in disease prevention and control.

Reducing the pain. Patients in treatment and examination often feel some discomfort. The discomfort may be caused by fear of hospital, or allergy to the instruments and equipment. In addition, patients while doing inspection are often in a state of high tension. Wearable devices can significantly improve the patient's clinic experience, because they can collect the data in an unconscious mannerly.

3.2   Wearable Medical Devices' "Weakness"

While wearable devices bring convenience to medical treatment, many problems also emerge. The Daily Mail reported that a non-profit organization named Open Effect and the University of Toronto has conducted a new study and found that popular fitness tracking devices on the market tend to disclose personal information [6]. Because the data collection is not restricted by time and place, the difficulty of data management and control increases. Privacy leak happens quite often. Equipment manufacturers including Fitbit, Garmin, Xiaomi, Withings and Jawbone, their devices were reported with the privacy problems. Some health medical wearable devices were forced to withdraw from the market for privacy reasons. Promulgated by the State Council in 2015, "the big data security system" and "strengthening security support" were both emphasized in "the notification about issuing the action program of promoting the development of large data [7]".

Data leakage of wearable device is mainly due to two reasons, the internal defects and external attacks. Internal vulnerabilities mainly refer to the equipment's defects in terms of software and hardware, which can be found out easily. Because of the products' independently, it is hard to patch or upgrade them. In addition, the open system is also a kind of internal defects. In general, with the method of the Bluetooth or wireless connection, wearable devices are easy to be invaded by hackers and lead to data leakage. External attacks mainly refer to some hackers' attempting to get data, usually by means of wireless attacks and malicious code.

Compared with the traditional medical mode, data collected by wearable devices has more opportunities to be attacked. The reasons may be the easy data acquisition methods, privacy more than content, using wireless network transmission, more data flow links, but without uniform data standards. Zhang Peijiang [8], Li Ruichang, Ma Bo [9], and Liu Jinfang et al. [10] considered that aspects such as vulnerabilities of Google android system, malicious software installation, the equipment's high dependence on unsafe mobile and wireless networks, may cause the wearable device data leakage.

3.3 Wearable Medical Devices' "Opportunities"

Target population growth. According to the United Nations population ageing standard, the world has entered the aging society. "Social old-age service system planning (2011–2015)", published in 2011 by the State Council, pointed out that the development of Chinese aging has speeded up. It is estimated that China will enter the stage of accelerated aging in 2020–2050. By the year 2050, as a result of the baby boom in the sixties and seventies of the last century, the aging population will reach 400 million and the aging level will reach 30% [11]. In addition, according to the "Chinese chronic disease prevention and control plan for 2012–2015", which was issued by the Ministry of Health in 2012, chronic diseases rejuvenation is becoming more and more serious. Deaths caused by chronic disease has accounted for 85% of the total death in our country. The disease burden caused by that has accounted for 70% of the total burden of disease [11]. Both long period of illness and large requirements indicate wearable devices will have a broad market in the field of medical treatment.

Investment boom springs up. According to data from the iMedia Re – search, 2012's China wearable equipment market scale is 420 million RMB, which is expected to reach 4.77 billion RMB in 2017, with compound annual growth rate of 60% [12]. According to the Swiss company Soreon study predicts that by 2020 the smart wearable device can help to save 1.3 million lives. According to "The wearable medical equipment market present situation analysis", which was issued by Cic advisory, scale of wearable medical equipment market of China in 2015 has already reached 1.19 billion RMB, and it is expected to exceed 2.37 billion RMB in 2016 [13]. Enterprises have also aimed at wearable medical market both at home and abroad. International enterprises, Qualcomm, Apple, Samsung, SONY, etc., all have invested in wearable medical market. Domestic companies, such as Danbond Technology, Ingenic, Andon Health, have released wearable products. In March 2014, the Blood Pressure Butler got a total of 10 million RMB investments from Grasp Hong Capital and North Soft Angel. In March 2014, Kangkang blood pressure got A round of investment of 30 million RMB from GuangmangVenture Capital Fund.

3.4 Wearable Medical Devices' "Threats"

Doubt of technical indicators. Data collected by wearable devices are multitudinous and interminable. The lack of professional guidance and inline standard leads to the low accuracy of the information. In most cases, the data collected by the wearable equipment is far from the clinical data. Some equipment is only a certain electronic products using medical technology rather than medical equipment. That is why they are not recognized by clinic doctors. Although the data are collected, however, they have no clinical value.

Lack of facility maintenance. To ensure its accuracy, the medical equipment in hospital will be maintained, verified and debugged periodically. Because of the high cost of equipment maintenance, most businesses will no longer provide free maintenance service after selling the products to patients. Patients will also no longer purchase the corresponding service for the same reason. As the growth of the service life, the accuracy of data collected by the equipment is questionable.

Hazard legal and moral. At present, there are no relevant laws and regulations, which specifically request the manufacturers of wearable devices to make sure that the data collected by the products should be close to the clinical data. But patients rely on these devices for a long time, believing in the data produced by these devices. If disease treatment was not in time, the responsibility of the problem is still not clear.

4 Revelation and Prospect

Once the concept of wearable medical devices was put forward, a great mass fervour of all circles in research and development is raised up. Technology is a double-edged sword. We should not only recognize that the wearable devices bring us assistance in the field of smart health, but should also be clear that wearable devices have the defects. We have to seize the opportunity in time, and cope with the challenge, then we can make full use of the benefits of good science and technology progress. Improvement and promotion of wearable devices still have a long way to go. Let's hope the application of wearable device can bring infinite possibility for medical wisdom.

References

1. Xu, G.: China's disease prevention and control work progress. Issued by National Health and Family Planning Commission of the People's Republic of China, report [EB/OL]. (2015). http://www.360doc.com/content/15/0421/10/20500003_464794906.shtml, Accessed 24 Apr 2015
2. Kirks, R.: Wearable devices-the future of individualized health care. Chin. Med. Manage. Sci. **1**, 34–37 (2016)
3. Yan, W.: Wearable medical devices have prospects, technology and capital is the short band. China Qual. J. **09**, 74–75 (2014)
4. The China securities network. Stanford new inventions to detonate wearable medical care and four stocks will start soon. http://www.gf.com.cn/cms/newsContent.jsp?docId=1807490. 2013-05-31
5. Intel Edison Chips. http://www.go-gddq.com/html/s628/2014-01/1223686.htm, Accessed 27 Jan 2014
6. Study shows most wearable devices will disclose personal information. http://www.cnbeta.com/articles/472775.htm, Accessed 04 Feb 2016
7. He, X., Qing, Q., Wu, S., Zhang, Z., Kong, X.: The study on the security and privacy of wearable device data in health care. Chin. Med. Books Intell. Mag. **10**, 32–37 (2016)
8. Zhang, P., Li, R.: Wearable computing application status and prospect in the field of medical and health care. In: China Information Research Institute of Chinese Medicine. Papers of the First Session of China's Traditional Chinese Medicine Information, p. 5 (2014)
9. Ma, B., He, X., Liu, X.: Wearable equipment development trend and the information security risk analysis. China's New Commun. **09**, 8 (2015)
10. Liu, J.: The information security risk of wearable devices and coping suggestions in our country. Inform. Secur. Technol. **11**, 10–12 (2014)
11. Wide prospect of wearable health medical equipment. Health Manage. **02**, 25–31 (2014)
12. Shang, Y., Sun, B.: The study on the status quo of smart health application under the background of big data. Sci. Technol. Ind. **10**, 19–27 (2016)
13. Cic advisory. Wearable medical equipment market present situation analysis [EB/OL]. http://wenku.baidu.com/link?url=AGSnAL3uXfOr676ix-OcwPh5MaTCGZSFiFHL-EzuQek_c_LFJ0pozErX7B2vaNbW6l4VD3fuLcUb0VbvIRJFRyWb84EP39WF8DBQ8MEepNK

A New Inverse Nth Gravitation Based Clustering Method for Data Classification

Huarong Xu$^{(\boxtimes)}$, Li Hao, Chengjie Jianag, and Ejaz Ul Haq

Department of Computer Science and Technology, Xiamen University of Technology,
Xiamen 361024, China
hrxu@xmut.edu.cn, {923752195,1181502446,ejaz4616}@qq.com

Abstract. Data classification is one of the core technologies in the field of pattern recognition and machine learning, which is of great theoretical significance and application value. With the increasing improvement of data acquisition, storage, transmission means and the amount of data, how to extract the essential attribute data from massive data, data accurate classification has become an important research topic. Inverse nth n order gravitational field is essentially a generalization of the n order in the physics, which can effectively describe the interaction between all the particles in the gravitational field. This paper proposes a new inverse nth power gravitation (I-n-PG) based clustering method is proposed for data classification. Some randomly generated data samples as well as some well-known classification data sets are used for the verification of the proposed I-n-PG classifier. The experiments show that our proposed I-n-PG classifier performs very well on both of these two test sets.

Keywords: Data classification · Inverse nth power gravitation · Clustering algorithm

1 Introduction

1.1 Background

With the rapid development of data acquisition, storage and transmission technology, the number of digital data storage is growing, which provides a wealth of information for the production and life of human. But at the same time, with the sharp increase in the amount of data, the human has not in limited time interested data were analyzed one by one, which gives the mankind put forward a new challenge, how to automatically achieve massive data classification by computer?

Data classification is one of the core technologies in pattern recognition and machine learning. It has been widely used in many aspects of people's production and life. The goal of data classification is to automatically extract the model from the known data set, and then judge the classification of unknown data. In recent years, researchers have carried out extensive research in data classification, put forward the classification method of large amounts of data, including decision tree classification method, Bayes method, classification method, classification based on neural network based

© Springer International Publishing AG 2017
C. Xing et al. (Eds.): ICSH 2016, LNCS 10219, pp. 9–18, 2017.
DOI: 10.1007/978-3-319-59858-1_2

classification method, subspace learning and manifold learning based on kernel learning classification method and so on. However, these methods still cannot fully reveal the mass data concentration the relationship between the data, so how to effectively describe the correlation between the data structure and has strong discriminative ability of the classifier, one of the problems to be solved is still facing researchers.

The inverse n^{th} [1–3] is a generalized n order generalized field in physics, which can effectively describe the interaction of all the particles in the gravitational field. In the gravitational field, each particle is subjected to the gravitational force of the other particles and is maintained in a state of dynamic equilibrium. Once a new particle to enter or exit the gravitational field, the dynamic balance of the original state will be broken, all the particles in the gravitational field will be in accordance with their respective force movement adjustment, finally realize the new dynamic balance. If each data set as an inverse n^{th} particle in gravitational field, and give it a certain quality in accordance with certain rules, then the data can be mapped to an inverse n^{th} gravitational field, the classification of the data will be transformed into the original particle in the field of inverse n^{th} gravity classification problem. The interaction between particles in the field through the research of inverse n^{th} order to construct particle classification model, will be more effective to describe the intrinsic attributes of the original data, realizes the automatic classification of massive data accurately.

2   Related Works

As the core problem in the field of pattern recognition and machine learning, data classification has been studied in recent decades. Through continuous exploration and research, researchers have made many important achievements in the research of data classification.

The basic principle of decision tree classification is to use the information gain search data set with the maximum amount of information in the field of information, and then set up a decision tree node [4–8]. Then a branch of the tree is established according to the different values of the attribute field, and the next node and the corresponding branch of each branch are continued to build the tree. Finally, each path in the decision tree corresponds to a rule, and the whole decision tree corresponds to a set of expression rules. For example, Murth gives a general procedure for constructing decision trees based on a given data set [5]. Zheng [7] presents a multi variable decision tree algorithm, which improves the classification accuracy of decision trees by constructing new binary features. Brazdil and Gama [8] fusion decision tree and linear discriminant model are used to construct multi variable decision tree. In this model, the new feature is obtained by the linear combination of the previous features.

The basic principle Bayes classification is to use probability to describe the data samples of the category of uncertainty, in the case of a priori probability and conditional probability is known, based on the Bayes theorem to predict the type of test samples [9–11]. In the literature, the existing Bayes classification methods can be divided into Naive Bayes classifiers [9] and Bayesian Networks [10, 11] two categories. Naive Bayes classifiers assume that each feature in a given feature is independent from each other. This assumption limits the scope of application of Naive Bayes classifiers, but its expression is simple and can effectively deal with the classification problem of independent (or approximately independent) features of some features. However, in many cases, the characteristics of the feature sets are often not independent, but have a strong correlation, the relationship between these features cannot be trained through the simple Bayes classifier. Bayes network is a graphical network based on probabilistic reasoning, which allows the definition of class conditional independence between subsets of variables, so it can effectively deal with the problem of data classification in feature correlation.

Artificial neural network classification [12–15]: artificial neural network is mathematical model that simulate neural network behavior characteristics and process distributed parallel information, has a wide range of applications in the pattern classification. Lain and Lee [15] analyses the use of artificial neural network to construct text classifier and dimensionality reduction method. Kon and Plaskota [13] studythe necessary minimum number of neurons in the feedforward neural network for a given task. Siddique and Tokhi [14] use genetic algorithm to train the weights of artificial neural network.

The classification based on spatial learning and manifold learning: In linear discriminant analysis (LDA) [31], the original high dimensional samples are projected into the low dimensional subspace, while ensuring the original sample with the maximum and minimum distance between class distance in low dimensional subspace. Dick et al. proposed a supervised locally linear embedding algorithm based on the original local linear embedding algorithm [27, 28], which can maintain the local topological relations of the original data in the low dimensional data. Tenenbaum et al. propose a manifold learning method (Isomap [29]) based on geodesic distance based on MDS (Scaling Multidimensional). Belkin and Niyogi proposed Laplacian Eigenmaps [30], whose basic idea is to use an undirected weighted graph to describe a manifold, and the low dimensional expression of the original sample is embedded in the graph. He et al. propose the Linearization of the method in the literature [30], and the Laplacian face [37] is proposed. The method is to keep the neighbor relationship between samples before and after dimensionality reduction. Yan et al. [38] proposed a unified framework for graph embedding based on the sample neighbor relationship, and an interval Fisher analysis method (MFA) was proposed

Kernel based classification [39, 40, 17–26]: the basic idea is to map the samples from low dimensional space to high dimensional feature space by kernel function. The linear non separable data samples in the input space can be linearly separable in the feature space with higher dimension. For example, Vapnik [25] proposed is to establish a learning kernel method based on statistical theory and support vector machine (Support Vector Machine, SVM), its basic principle is to find a optimal classification requirements of the hyperplane, the hyperplane in ensuring the precision of classification at the same time, the maximum over both sides of the plane interval. In theory, the support vector machine is able to achieve the optimal classification of linear separable data. Tipping [41] put forward the relevance vector machine (Relevance Vector Machine, RVM), its basic principle is the point of decision theory to remove irrelevant structure in active correlation based on priori parameters, to obtain the sparse model. How to select a suitable kernel function based on the kernel function classification method is not suitable for a given data set.

Classification based on sparse representation: a face recognition method based on sparse representation is proposed by [34]. This method assumes that the face image can be represented as a linear combination of a small number of samples in the training data set. Based on the same assumption, the paper proposed a method of facial image restoration and recognition based on sparse representation [35]. Using the sparsity of wavelet coefficients, a new method of wavelet denoising based on sparse representation is proposed in the paper, which is based on the [36]. Although the sparse representations in many classification applications show excellent performance, however, recently, there are some references [31–33] further discuss the role of sparse representation plays in the image classification problem of face recognition.

3   The New Gravitation Based Clustering Algorithm

A new data clustering approach based on inverse nth power gravitation for large scale data classification is present in this section. Before the discussion of the new algorithm, we firstly discuss some knowledge about the universal gravitation.

The traditional law of gravitation was proposed by Newton in 1687, with the equation shown below in Eq. 1, where F is the force, G is the gravitational constant ($G = 6.67 * 10 - 11$), m1 and m2 are the masses of the object interacting, r is the distance between the centers of the masses.

$$F = G \times \frac{m_1 \times m_2}{r^2} \tag{1}$$

This gravitation is everywhere, and gravitation also shows effect on space-time such as distortion generated by the mass of an object in general relativity. A figure of this distortion is shown below in Fig. 1.

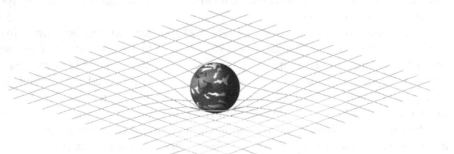

Fig. 1. Space-time distortion affected by gravitation

Gravitation not only can make distortion over space-time, but also can be utilized for data clustering. Samples in each training set can be considered as particles, and if each particle is assigned a mass value, then we can form a new attraction equation. We make an extension of the traditional equation of gravitation shown in Eq. 1 to a new one, shown in Eq. 2

$$F(x_i, x_j) = \frac{m(x_i)m(x_j)}{\left\|x_i - x_j\right\|^{n+1}}(x_i - x_j), n \geq 2 \tag{2}$$

X_i and X_j are two D-dimensional samples/particles in the training set with the mass values $m(X_i)$ and $m(X_j)$. We denote the equation as the inverse nth power gravitation (I-n-PG) for data classification. The mass values of X_i and X_j incorporate the gravitational constant G, so there is no G in Eq. 2.

For the training set S,S $= \{x_1, x_2, \ldots, x_N\} \subset R^D$, there are N samples in it. As to each sample X of set S in the gravitation field, the attraction force can be calculated by Eq. 3.

$$F(S, x) = m(x) \sum_{x_i \in S} \frac{m(x_i)}{\left\|x_i - x\right\|^{n+1}}(x_i - x) \tag{3}$$

Accordingly, modulo of F(S, x) can be calculated according to Eq. 4.

$$F_m(S, x) = \|F(S, x)\| = m(x)\| \sum_{x_i \in S} \frac{m(x_i)}{\left\|x_i - x\right\|^{n+1}}(x_i - x)\| \tag{4}$$

The flowchart of the new proposed I-n-PG large scale data classification algorithm can be illustrated as follows (Fig. 2):

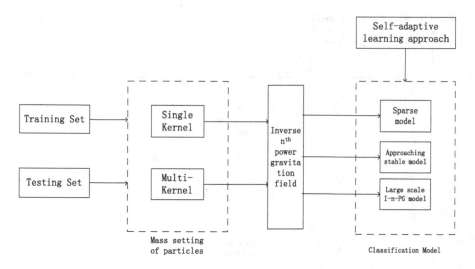

Fig. 2. The flowchart of the I-n-PG model

For the assignment of particle mass value of X_i, a kernel learning based approach is proposed. There are mainly two approaches, one is based on single kernel, and the other is on multi-kernel. In the single kernel approach, samples are projected into high dimensional space by kernel function, the mass value of a certain particle X_i in inverse n^{th} gravitation field can be calculated by the neighborhood distance of the particle in the kernel space. The nearer the distance toward other samples in the same class is, the heavier the particle mass is. Training samples and proper kernel function are used for the parameters adaption, and then we can calculate the mass value of particles. In the multi-kernel approach, it is an enhancement of the single kernel approaching, and it is used for tackling the cases that the training samples are in large scales, and usually are heterogeneous, that the single kernel approach cannot tackle. The multi-kernel model are constructed as follows in Eq. 5.

$$K = \sum_{i=1}^{M} \alpha_i K_i \qquad (5)$$

Where, $\alpha_i \geq 0, \sum_{i-1}^{M} \alpha_i = 1$, K_i denotes the ith kernel function, M is the number of kernels. Then Mass value of particles are calculated by the neighborhood distance in the multi-kernel space. Figure 3 gives the illustration of the calculation of mass value of certain particle in multi-kernel space.

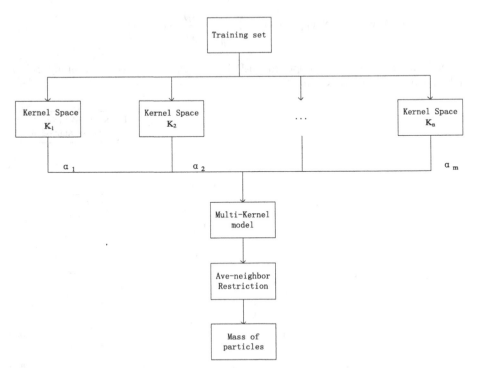

Fig. 3. The Mass value calculation in multi-kernel space

For the steady state calculation in the gravitational field, if a particle in the field has a relative small attraction force, it is considered as in a steady state, and when 90% of the particles in the training set are in steady state, we supposed this case a steady state of the particles. The new I-n-PG classifier can be illustrated as follows in Fig. 4.

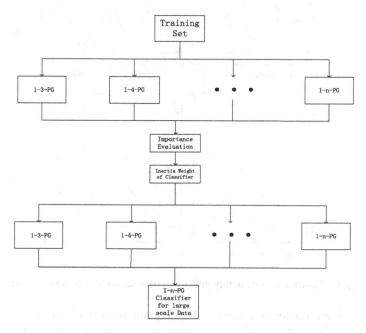

Fig. 4. The new I-N-PG classifier for large scale data

4 Experiment Result Analysis

Randomly generated data set as well as a well-known classification data set, the IRIS data are used here for the verification of the proposed inverse nth gravitation based classifier. Several well-known clustering approaches such as 1NN, SVM SGF network are also used for the comparison here. For the randomly generated data of 2dimension samples, figures are given for the classification of different data samples.

Figure 5 gives the classification results by the I-n-PG classifier in a 2-D data set. The classification process begins the mass values initialization of samples in the nth gravitation field, and then the calculation of steady state are done over all these samples. Then, the I-n-PG classifier are constructed based single kernel approach or multi-kernel approach. Finally, samples are classified by the I-n-PG classifier. In Fig. 5.

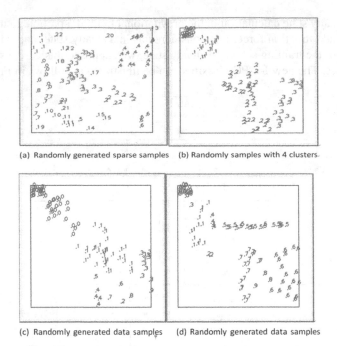

(a) Randomly generated sparse samples   (b) Randomly samples with 4 clusters

(c) Randomly generated data samples   (d) Randomly generated data samples

Fig. 5. Illustration of randomly generated data set under I-n-PG classifier

(a) samples are randomly generated in a square space without evident clusters. Samples in Fig. 5(b) can be easily seen that there are four clusters. Figure 5(c) gives samples with two evident clusters while other samples are in sparse and randomly locations. Figure 5(d) shows some lines cluster cases. Table 1 gives the comparison between the proposed I-n-PG classifier and some well-known classifiers, 1NN, SVM and SGF network under IRIS data sets. We can see form the table that the classic 1NN classifier achieves 94.2% success, classic SVM achieves 97.4% success, SGF network secure same performance as SVM classifier, and the proposed I-n-PG classifier outperforms all these contrasted ones.

Table 1. Comparison of best result for IRIS data set

I-n-PG	1NN	SVM	SGF network
98.5%	94.2%	97.4%	97.4%

5 Conclusion

In this paper, new inverse n^{th} power gravitation (I-n-PG) based clustering method is proposed for data classification. Some randomly generated data samples as well as some well-known classification data sets are used for the verification of the proposed I-n-PG classifier. The experiments show that our proposed I-n-PG classifier performs very well on both of these two test sets. A future work is to reduce the time cost during the classification process as the calculation of nth distance and the adaptive parameter for the steady state consumes lots of time.

Acknowledgment. This work was supported by National Nature Science Foundation of China under the research project 61273290.

References

1. Chandrasekhar, S.: Newton's Principia for the Common Reader. Oxford University Press, New York (1995)
2. Heintz, W.H.: Runge-Lenz vector for non- relativistic Kepler motion modified by an inverse cube force. Am. J. Phys. **44**(7), 687–694 (1976)
3. Roseveare, N.: Mercury's Perihelion from Le verrier to Einstein. Oxford University Press, New York (1982)
4. Paul, E.: Incremental Induction of Decision Trees. Mach. Learn. **4**(2), 161–186 (1997)
5. Murthy, S.K.: Automatic construction of decision trees from data: a multi-disciplinary survey. Data Min. Knowl. Disc. **2**, 345–389 (1998)
6. Mugambi, E.M.: Polynomial—fuzzy data knowledge-based systems: decision tree structures for classifying medical data. Knowl.-Based Syst. **17**(2), 81–87 (2004)
7. Zheng, Z.: Constructing conjunctions using systematic search on decision trees. Knowl. Based Syst. J. **10**, 421–430 (1998)
8. Gama, J., Brazdil, P.: Linear Tree. Intell. Data Anal. **3**, 1–22 (1999)
9. Meretakis, D., Wuthrieh, B.: Extending Naive Bayes classifiers using long itemsets. In: Proceeding 1999 International Conference Knowledge Discovery and Data Mining (KDD 1999), San Diego, pp. 165–174, August 1999
10. Cheng, J., Bell, D., Liu, W.: Learning Bayesian Networks from Data: An Efficient Approach Based on Information Theory (1999)
11. Acid, S., de Campos, L.M.: Searching for Bayesian Network structures in the space of restricted acyclic partially directed graphs. J. Artif. Intell. Res. **18**, 445–490 (2003)
12. Zhang, G.: Neural networks for classification: a survey. IEEE Trans. Syst. Man Cybern. Part C **30**(4), 451–462 (2000)
13. Kon, M., Plaskota, L.: Information complexity of neural networks. Neural Netw. **13**, 365–375 (2000)
14. Siddique, M.N.H., Tokhi, M.O.: Training neural networks: backpropagation vs. genetic algorithms. In: IEEE International Joint Conference on Neural Networks, vol. 4, pp. 2673–2678 (2011)
15. Lam Savio, L.Y., Lee, D.L.: Feature reduction for neural network based text categorization. In: Digital Symposium Collection of 6th International Conference on Database System for Advanced Application (1999)
16. Ji, S.W., Xu, W., Yang, M., Yu, K.: 3D convolutional neural networks for human action recognition. In: The 27th International Conference on Machine Learning, pp. 495–502 (2010)
17. Damoulas, T., Girolami, M.A.: Pattern Recognition with a Bayesian Kernel Combination Machine (2009)
18. Kingsbury, N., Tay, D.B.H., Palaniswami, M.: Multi-Scale Kernel Methods for Classification (2005)
19. Li, B., Zheng, D., Sun, L.: Exploiting Multi-Scale Support Vector Regression for Image Compression (2007)

20. Pozdnoukhov, A., Kanevski, M.: Multi-Scale Support Vector Algorithms for Hot Spot Detection and Modeling (2007)
21. Lin, Y.Y., Liu, T.L., Fuh, C.S.: Local Ensemble Kernel Learning for Object Category Recognition (2007)
22. Sonnenburg, S., Rlitsch, G., Schafer, C.: A General and Efficient Multiple Kernel Learning Algorithm (2005)
23. Smola, A.J., SchOlkopf, B.: A Tutorial on Support Vector Regression (2004)
24. Vapnik, V.N.: The Nature of Statistical Learning Theory. Springer, New York (1995)
25. Karampatziakis, N.: Static analysis of binary executables using structural SVMs. Adv. Neural. Inf. Process. Syst. **23**, 1063–1071 (2010)
26. Ridder, D., Kouropteva, O., Okun, O., Pietikäinen, M., Duin, Robert P.W.: Supervised locally linear embedding. In: Kaynak, O., Alpaydin, E., Oja, E., Xu, L. (eds.) ICANN/ICONIP -2003. LNCS, vol. 2714, pp. 333–341. Springer, Heidelberg (2003). doi:10.1007/3-540-44989-2_40
27. Roweis, S.T., Saul, L.K.: Nonlinear dimensionality reduction by locally linear embedding. Science **290**, 2323–2326 (2000)
28. Tenenbaum, J.B., de Silva, V., Langford, J.C.: A global geometric framework for nonlinear dimensionality reduction. Science **290**, 2319–2323 (2000)
29. Belkin, M., Niyogi, P.: Laplacian Eigen maps for dimensionality reduction and data representation. Neural Comput. **15**(6), 1373–1396 (2003)
30. Rigamonti, R., Brown, M., Lepetit, V.: Are sparse representation really relevant for image classification? In: Proceeding of International Conference on Computer Vision and Pattern Recognition (2011)
31. Shi, Q., Eriksson, A., Van Den Hengel, A., Shen, C.: Is face recognition really a Compressive Sensing problem? In: Proceeding of International Conference on Computer Vision and Pattern Recognition (2011)
32. Zhang, L., Yang, M., Feng, X.: Sparse representation or collaborative representation: which helps face recognition? In: Proceeding of International Conference on Computer Vision (2011)
33. Wright, J., Yang, A.Y., Ganesh, A., Sastry, S.S., Ma, Y.: Robust face recognition via sparse representation. PAMI **31**(2), 210–227 (2009)
34. Zhang, H., Yang, J., Zhang, Y., Huang, T.: Close the loop: joint blind image restoration and recognition with sparse representation prior. In: ICCV (2011)
35. He, X., Yan, S., Hu, Y., Niyogi, P., Zhang, H.J.: Face recognition using Laplacianfaces. IEEE Trans. Pattern Anal. Mach. Intell. **27**(3), 328–340 (2005)
36. Yan, S., Dong, X., Zhang, B., Zhang, H., Yang, Q., Lin, S.: Graph embedding and extensions: a general framework for dimensionality reduction. IEEE Trans. Pattern Anal. Mach. Intell. **29**(1), 40–51 (2007)
37. Lanckriet, G.R.G., Cristianini, N., Bartlett, P., Ghaoui, L.E., Jordan, M.I.: Learning the kernel matrix with semidenite programming. J. Mach. Learn. Res. **5**(1), 27–72 (2004)
38. Lee, W.-J., Verzakov, S., Duin, R.P.W.: Kernel combination versus classifier combination. In: Haindl, M., Kittler, J., Roli, F. (eds.) MCS 2007. LNCS, vol. 4472, pp. 22–31. Springer, Heidelberg (2007). doi:10.1007/978-3-540-72523-7_3
39. Tipping, M.E.: The relevance vector machine. In: Proceeding of Advances in Neural Information Processing Systems, vol. 12, pp. 652–658 (2000)

Extracting Clinical-event-packages
from Billing Data for Clinical Pathway Mining

Haowei Huang, Tao Jin$^{(\boxtimes)}$, and Jianmin Wang

Key Laboratory for Information System Security, Ministry of Education,
Tsinghua National Laboratory for Information Science and Technology,
School of Software, Tsinghua University, Beijing 100084, China
huanghw10@gmail.com, jintao05@gmail.com, jimwang@tsinghua.edu.cn

Abstract. Clinical pathway can be used to reduce medical cost and improve medical efficiency. Traditionally, clinical pathways are designed by experts based on their experience. However, it is time consuming and sometimes not adaptive for specific hospitals, and mining clinical pathways from historic data can be helpful. Clinical pathway naturally can be regarded as a kind of process, and process mining can be used for clinical pathway mining. However, due to the *complexity* and *dynamic* of medical behaviors, traditional process mining methods often generate spaghetti-like clinical pathways with too many nodes and edges. To reduce the number of nodes in the resulting models, we put correlated events into *clinical-event-packages* as new units of log event for further mining. The experiment results has shown that our approach is a good way of generating more comprehensible clinical process as well as packages with better quality according to medical practitioners.

Keywords: Clinical-event-package · Process mining · Clinical process

1   Introduction

Clinical pathways (CP), also known as care pathways, is used as one of the main tools for quality management as well as expense control and resource regulation in healthcare. Experiments have proved that the implementation of CP reduces the variability in clinical practice and improves outcomes.

In China, more than 300 CPs has been implemented since 2009 in order to standardize care processes in hospitals and in turn to bring down the medical expenses. However, most of the CPs used in hospitals or released by government are designed by experts based on their experience, which can be lack of data support in the perspective of evidence-based medicine (EBM). What's more, today's hospital information systems contain a wealth of data as the volume of healthcare-related data growing dramatically with the increasing use of electronic health record systems (EHR), picture archiving and communication systems (PACS), and many more systems that collect data. It will be of great help if we could extract clinical pathways out of past clinical data and provide the doctors and experts with data support and refine existing clinical pathways.

© Springer International Publishing AG 2017
C. Xing et al. (Eds.): ICSH 2016, LNCS 10219, pp. 19–31, 2017.
DOI: 10.1007/978-3-319-59858-1_3

As clinical process is a good way to present clinical pathways, we can use the techniques of process mining [1] to mine the workflow of clinical activities from the clinical logs. However, due to the dynamic and complexity of medical behaviors in clinical data, existing process mining techniques either generate spaghetti-like clinical pathway models that are incomprehensible to people, or usually discover excessive volume of clinical pathway models such that the meanings or significance of the discovered clinical pathway models sometimes goes untold. How to derive clinical processes using process mining technologies remains a great challenge.

In this paper, a novel approach for reducing the scale of different clinical events in clinical data is presented by putting related events into *clinical-event-packages* as new units of log event for further mining, which allows us to use traditional process mining toolkits as well as algorithms unimpededly. Depending on this idea we proposed an approach of clinical process mining. As illustrated in Fig. 2, the pipeline consists of three parts, Data Preprocessing, Clinical-event-package Discovery and Clinical process Mining. The major achievements of this paper is in the second stage, we introduce a pioneering two-level strategy named *CEPM* to extract *clinical-event-packages* by finding *co-occurrence* activities.

The main contributions of our work are:

- We propose a feasible way to apply traditional process mining techniques on clinical data by putting correlate events into packages as new units of log event to reduce the number of different clinical events.
- To the best of our knowledge, our packing method CEPM is the first work that uses the co-occurrence relation based on conditional probability to generate packages of events.
- A 2-level packing strategy is implemented in our packing method that can help us get more accurate packages.

The remainder of this paper is organized as follows. In Sect. 2 we briefly review the related work. Section 3 gives introduction to our dataset and some preliminaries about clinical event. Our method of clinical process mining as well as our packing strategy CEPM will be presented in Sect. 4. Experimental results and analysis will be given in Sect. 5. Section 6 concludes the paper and sketches the future work.

2   Related Work

The exploration of medical knowledge from clinical data (mostly EMRs) with data mining techniques is an important problem that has been the focus of study on recent medical informatics research. In general, there are two orientations of studies: *holistic* and *localized*.

The goal of a *holistic* study is to explore knowledge that can describe the overall event traces of the patient population. The typical techniques of this kind are process mining techniques, as they can discover the process model by inferring the ordering relations between various tasks in the event log.

Lang et al. [3] reached the conclusion in their research that traditional process mining approaches had problems dealing with unstructured processes from medical environments, as they did a detailed hands-on evaluation and analysis of seven classic process mining approaches[1] and concluded that none of the discussed approaches was able to meet all major challenges of mining clinical processes.

To avoid the clutter caused by *holistic* studies, *localized* studies focus more on exploring the local characteristics of the patient event traces. For example, Gotz et al. [4] constructed a strategy to mining frequent pattern within time intervals, where they build an interactive visual framework for doctors. A doctor first selects patient trace segments by giving time nodes, the system will then mine frequent patterns out of the selected data using a bitmap-base mining algorithm named SPAM [5] and a visual output of these patterns will be given at last. Huang et al. [6] proposed a novel approach to mine closed clinical pathway patterns from event log. Although it surpasses general sequence pattern mining algorithms in many ways, there are still a number of infrequent behaviors that are missing in the discovered patterns while these infrequent behaviors can be very important in clinical pathways and should not be missed. Zhang et al. [7] used hierarchical clustering based on longest common subsequence (LCS) distance to discover six patient subgroups and derived common clinical pathways for each subgroup by based on probabilities, while the interpretability of each clinical pathways still has some defects. Perer et al. [8] adapted a frequent sequence mining algorithm to handle the real-world properties of EMR data. During their work they find the phenomenon which they call *pattern explosion* that caused a great challenge for frequent pattern mining algorithms, as they detect patterns with all possible combinations of events and subsets of events occurring at the same time. So in the data preprocessor, they used frequent itemset mining technique Apriori [10] to detect frequent Clinical Event Packages as super events. Yet the resulted packages are still used for further frequent pattern mining rather than process mining.

In conclusion, it is a solid fact that the diversity of medical behaviors and the complexity of chronicle information among medical behaviors in clinical process far surpasses that of common business processes, and both traditional process mining techniques and frequent pattern mining strategies are facing great challenges in the exploration of medical knowledge. Thus, the innovation of mining approaches is necessary and important.

3   Preliminaries

In this section, we will introduce the basis of billing data and define related concepts and giving examples.

---

[1] These seven approaches are the α algorithm, the α++ algorithm, the Heuristic mining algorithm, the DWS-algorithm, the multiphase-algorithm, the genetic miner, and theory-of-regions-based algorithm.

3.1   Billing Data Basis

There are three levels of data in the hierarchy of clinical data in China, i.e., the *billing data, medical order* and *clinical pathway form-item* form bottom to top. Among them clinical pathway in the top level is more like a guidance and what we can get from the Electronic Medical Record (EMR) system are billing data and medical order records. Here we choose the billing data as the raw data rather than the medical order records because it is more detailed and contains more information, and medical order can sometimes be abstract and may not be easy to understand.

Table 1. A sample of billing data

Patient ID	Activity	Category	Time stamp
1	Level I care	Nursing fee	8/21/2011
1	CBC	Pathological examination fee	8/22/2011
1	Intravenous infusion	Treatment cost	8/22/2011
2	X-ray computed tomography	Nursing fee	3/11/2012
2	Glycerol fructose	Western medicine cost	3/11/2012

On the level of billing data, the EMRs record every single item a patient was charged during his/her stay in the hospital. In the dataset each record has a unique patient ID and an activity, along with a corresponding list of informations of the activity, for example, the time stamp, the category[2] and the charge of the activity, etc. Based on the focus of this paper, four properties of a record are concerned if we regard a record as a clinical event, and they are: (1) patient id, (2) activity, (3) category and (4) time stamp (accurate to the day). As shown in Table 1, each line refers to a clinical event.

3.2   Clinical Event Log

In this section, we will give definitions as well as examples of *clinical event log* related concepts.

Definition 1 (Clinical activity). *An activity a is the name of a clinical event. And we denote A as the activity domain, i.e. the set of all possible activities.*

Definition 2 (Clinical event). *Let ε be the clinical event universe, i.e., the set of all possible clinical events, PID be the patient identifier domain, A be the activity domain, C be the event category domain, and T the time domain.*

---

[2] The categories of activities of billing data are standardized by national specification, for example, there are 14 categories in our dataset: "checking free", "medicine costs", "checkups fee", "blood test fee", "pathological examination fee", "surgery fee", "anesthesia fee", "nursing fee", "heating fee", "bedding fee", "treatment cost", "western medicine cost", "supplies of special fees", and "other expenses".

clinical event log   patient trace   day trace

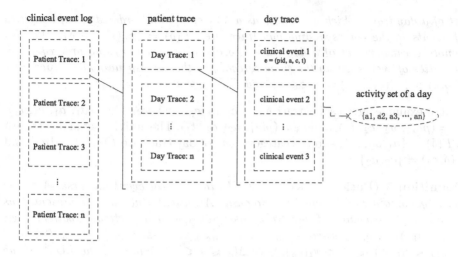

Fig. 1. Hierarchy of clinical event log related concepts

Formally, we use the functions $\pi_{pid} : \varepsilon \to PID$, $\pi_a : \varepsilon \to A$, $\pi_c : \varepsilon \to C$, and $\pi_t : \varepsilon \to T$ to denote the patient identifiers, the activity, the event category, and the time-stamps of clinical events, respectively.

For convenience, we denote a clinical event e as $e = (pid, a, c, t)$, where pid is the patient identifier of e ($pid \in PID$), a is the activity of e ($a \in A$), and t is the time stamp of e ($t \in T$). Taking Table 1 as an example, there is a specific clinical event $e = (1, \text{ } level \text{ } I \text{ } care, \text{ } nursing \text{ } fee, \text{ } 8/21/2011)$ where $\pi_{pid} = 1$ is the patient identifier, $\pi_a = level \text{ } I \text{ } care$ is the activity, $\pi_c = nursing \text{ } fee$ is the event category, and $\pi_t = 8/21/2011$ is the time stamp of e.

A *clinical event*, which represents a real-life clinical activity corresponding to a piece of record of billing data, is the basic unit of clinical event log, as shown in Table 1.

Definition 3 (Day trace). *Let ε be the clinical event universe, A be the activity domain and T the time domain. A day trace is represented as a non-empty sequence of events associated with a particular patient in a particular day of therapy, i.e., $\delta = \text{ } < e_1, e_2, ..., e_n >$, where $\pi_{pid}(e_1) \equiv \pi_{pid}(e_2) \equiv ... \equiv \pi_{pid}(e_n)$ and $\pi_t(e_1) \equiv \pi_t(e_2) \equiv ... \equiv \pi_t(e_n), e_i \in \varepsilon(1 \leqslant i \leqslant n)$. Let Δ be the day trace universe, and we use the functions $\pi_{pid} : \Delta \to PID$ and $\pi_t : \Delta \to T$ to denote the patient identifiers and the time-stamps of day traces, respectively.*

Definition 4 (Activity set and category set of a day trace).[3] *Let A be the activity domain, C be the event category domain, and $\Gamma(\delta)$ be the activity*

---

[3] We define these two concepts for the reason that for a given day trace we do not know the exact order of that each event happens (the order given by the system is surely unreliable), so we assume that the repeat of activities on a day should be removed and that we sort the sets under a unified standard.

set of a day trace, which we denote as a non-empty and ordered set of activities of events in the corresponding day trace, i.e., $\Gamma(\delta) = \{\pi_a(e)|e \in \delta\}$. We also denote a category set of a day trace $\Gamma(\delta, c)$ is a non-empty and ordered set of activities of events within the same category in the corresponding day trace, i.e., $\Gamma(\delta, c) = \{\pi_a(e)|\pi_c(e) = c,\ e \in \delta\}$ and $\Gamma(\delta, c)$ is a subset of $\Gamma(\delta)$.

For example, given a day trace $\delta = <e_1, e_2, e_3>$, where $e_1 = (pid_1, a_1, c_1, t_1)$, $e_2 = (pid_1, a_2, c_2, t_1)$, and $e_3 = (pid_1, a_3, c_2, t_1)$. The activity set of day trace δ is $\Gamma(\delta) = \{a_1, a_2, a_3\}$, and the category sets of day trace are $\Gamma(\delta, c_1) = \{a_1\}$ and $\Gamma(\delta, c_2) = \{a_2, a_3\}$.

Definition 5 (Patient trace). *Let ε be the clinical event universe, A be the activity domain and T the time domain. A patient trace σ is represented as a non-empty sequence of day traces associated with a particular patient, i.e., $\sigma = <\delta_1, \delta_2, ..., \delta_n>$, where $\pi_{pid(\delta_1)} \equiv \pi_{pid(\delta_2)} \equiv \cdots \equiv \pi_{pid(\delta_n)} = \pi_{pid}(\sigma)$, and $\pi_t(\delta_1) < \pi_t(\delta_2) < \cdots < \pi_t(\delta_n), \delta_i \in \Delta(1 \leqslant i \leqslant n)$, and n is the LOS[4] of the patient.*

Definition 6 (Clinical event log). *Let P be the set of all possible patient traces, and a clinical event log L is a set of patient traces, i.e., $L = \{\sigma_1, \sigma_2, ..., \sigma_n\}$, where $\sigma_i \in P$.*

The relationship between the above concepts are shown in Fig. 1.

4   Method

In this section we will explain our method of mining clinical process out of billing data especially our clinical event packing strategy in details, following the order of the pipeline shown in Fig. 2.

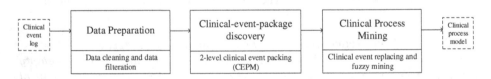

Fig. 2. The pipeline of CEPM based clinical process mining

4.1   Data Preparation

In the data preparation section, some data cleaning work is necessary in order to get rid of as much interference as possible and hopefully we can get a dataset with higher quality as the input of further works.

Firstly, we remove the redundant properties of clinical events and merge activities with homogeneous phrase. For example, we put phrases like "calcium

---

[4] LOS: length of stay in the hospital.

assay (colorimetry)" and "calcium assay (ISE)" together as one single activity called "calcium assay", and by doing this we reduced the number of different activities from 762 to 667 by 12.5%.

Secondly, we removed the record data of irrelevant categories. For example, "heating fee" and "bedding fee" are removed in the experiments in Sect. 5, because items in these two categories provide little medical information, however they may create interference during later process.

4.2   Clinial-event-package Discovery

We will first give the definition of two kind of relations before we go deep into the algorithm.

Definition 7 (Conditional probability of activities). *Let A be the clinical activity domain, and Δ be the day trace domain of all the day traces of a event log. The conditional probability of activity a_1 given activity a_2 is defined as $P(a_1|a_2) = \frac{N(a_1a_2)}{N(a_2)}$, where $N(a_2)$ is the number of day traces whose activity set contains a_2 $(a_2 \in \Gamma(\delta))$ and $N(a_1a_2)$ is the number of day traces whose activity set contains both a_1 and a_2 $(a_1, a_2 \in \Gamma(\delta))$.*

Definition 8 (Co-occurrence of two activities). *Let A be the clinical activity domain. Given two activities a_1 and $a_2 \in A$, and a minimum support threshold min_sup, we say a_1 and a_2 are co-occurrence on min_sup if both of the conditional probability $P(a_1|a_2)$ and $P(a_2|a_1)$ are greater than or equal to min_sup, i.e., $P(a_1|a_2) \geqslant min\_sup$ and $P(a_2|a_1) \geqslant min\_sup$.*

Definition 9 (Co-occurrence of two packages). *Given two packages pkg_1 and $pkg_2 \in PKG$, and a minimum support threshold min_sup, we say pkg_1 and pkg_2 are co-occurrence on min_sup if for $\forall a_1 \in pkg_1, a_2 \in pkg_2$, a_1 and a_2 are co-occurrence on min_sup.*

We believe that co-occurrence is a good character to describe the *relationship between two activities* as it can reflect how close and correlated they are, especially when the min_sup is set to a rather high value. In our experiment we choose 0.8 as the min_sup for the following reasons. On one hand, two activities that are co-occurrence on 0.8 can be regarded as highly correlated as each of them happens on no less than 80% of the cases when the other happens. On the other hand, setting the min_sup to 0.8 is under the consideration of dealing with the dynamic and flexibility of clinical data that we should improve the *Tolerance* of our method, which will be fully explained in Sect. 5.2. A clinical-event-package in our case is a set of activities in which every activity in it is co-occurrence on a certain min_sup to one another, and the two-level CEPM algorithm is designed to find these packages, as shown in Algorithm 1[5].

---

[5] Due to space limitations, we only illustrate the main structure of the CEPM algorithm here.

Algorithm 1. CLINICAL EVENT PACKAGE MINING (CEPM)

Input : L is a clinical event log

min_sup_c is the minimun support threshold for category level packing

min_sup_p is the minimun support threshold for patient level packing

Output: PS: a set of packages

1 Let C be the set of 12 categories L

2 Let D be the set of activity sets $\Gamma(\delta)$ of all the day traces in L

3 $PS_c \leftarrow$ new set of packages // the result of category-level packing

4 **for** *each* $c \in C$ **do**

5   Let $D(c)$ be the set of category sets $\Gamma(\delta, c)$ of all the day traces in L

6      $ps \leftarrow Packing(D(c),\ min\_sup_c)$

7   **for** *each set* $s \in ps$ **do**

8   add s to PS_c

9 Let L_n be the new event log after replacing event with packages in PS_c;

10 Let D_n be the set of activity sets $\Gamma(\delta)$ of all the day traces in L_n

11 $PS \leftarrow Packing(D_n,\ min\_sup_p)$

12 **return** PS

The input of our method is an event log L, and it will be transformed into a set of the activity sets (namely D) before it can be used as input of our packing algorithm. We use a two-level packing strategy in our method. First, we take advantage of the category information and extract packages within each categories by getting the set of *category sets* (Definition 4) of all the *day traces* in L (line 6 in Algorithm 1), and we use the *Packing* algorithm to extract packages within each category (line 3–8 in Algorithm 1) and replace the original events with these packages and we get a new event log, i.e., nL. In the *Packing* algorithm we use an incremental way of merging *co-occurrence* (Definition 9) packages to construct clinical-event-packages. Finally, we get the set of *activity sets* (namely D) of all the *day traces* in nL, by applying the *Packing* algorithm again on D (line 11 in Algorithm 1) we get the packages we want.

4.3   Clinical Process Mining

After we get all the packages, we will do some package filter work. First, we will remove the interference packages that only has one activity in it and appears only a couple of times in all day traces. Then, we select the most important packages for process mining by ranking the packages according to frequency among day traces and choose the top-20 packages with over 98% of *Patient Trace Coverage*[6]. After all this work we replace events with the packages we selected and use process mining algorithms to mine clinical process from the new event log.

---

[6] Patient Trace Coverage of an activity/package is the percentage of patients that the activity (package) was executed during his/her therapy among all patients.

So far we have explained the whole process of our method and the result will be discussed in Sect. 5.

5   Experiment Evaluation

In this section, we will evaluate our method in two aspects:

- On the level of Process. We set up an experiment to test if we can derive readable and comprehensible clinical process along our pipeline with traditional process mining algorithms as in Sect. 5.1.
- On the level of Packing strategy. Two experiments are implemented in this part, one is a comparison on the packing results between our method CEPM and another packing strategy based on Apriori algorithm in frequent itemset mining (Sect. 5.2), and the other is the comparison between strategies with and without the category level packing in CEPM (Sect. 5.3).

The dataset we are using in this work is the billing data of 240 patients with the disease *brain hemorrhage* from X hospital in the Y province of China. It is composed of 137254 billing data records which cover over 5 years of total time duration and 762 different activities of events belonging to 14 different categories from these 240 patients.

5.1   Evaluation on Clinical Process Mining

Along the pipeline shown in Fig. 2, we get 667 different activities from 12 categories after data preparation, and we get 65 packages as the result of CEPM algorithm with the min_sup of packing on both levels set to 0.8 and after removing the interference packages[7], then we select top-20 packages with over 98% of patient trace coverage as the input for process mining on toolkit Disco [9]. The Disco miner is based on the Fuzzy miner [2] which was the first mining algorithm to introduce the *map metaphor* to process mining, including advanced features like seamless process simplification and highlighting of frequent activities and paths, and it is a good choice for mining clinical process. And the resulting process model is shown in Fig. 3.

The process model reflects the most common treatment process of patients with cerebral hemorrhage, as shown in Fig. 3, each node refers to a package[8] with case frequency. We can see clearly from the workflow that when a patient first arrives in, he/she will first do a "x-ray computed tomography" to diagnose disease, which we mark as the first stage as shown in Fig. 3. Once diagnosed with *cerebral hemorrhage*, the patient becomes an in-patient and will enter the second stage during which he/she will be experiencing a series of test like "ambulatory blood pressure monitoring" with medicines like "compound chuanxiong capsule"

---

[7] As mentioned in Sect. 4.1, the interference packages are packages that only has one event in it and appears only a couple of times in all event traces.

[8] Some of them are listed in Fig. 4(b) in detail.

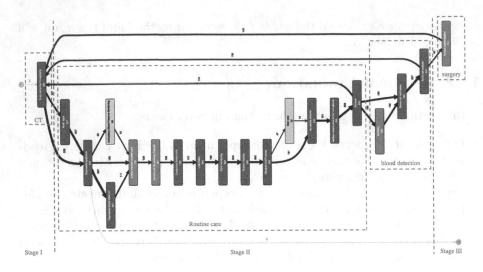

Fig. 3. The process model mined by Fuzzy Miner in Disco

and "compound amino acid" as well as essential nursing like "level I care". After all of this the doctor will run a series of blood test ("oximetry", etc.) to see if the patient is ready to move on to the third stage where an operation called "venous catheterization" will be executed and a following "x-ray computed tomography" will be done to detect if the patient is cured and is ready to discharge from hospital.

Since the whole process has been approved by medical practitioners we have the reason to believe that our method combined with Fuzzy miner can derive in a readable and comprehensible process model.

5.2 Evaluation on the Packing Result of CEPM

Traditional mining methods, for instance, the frequent itemset mining algorithms, are more frequently used in previous research for mining frequent patterns. In order to test the effectiveness of our method, i.e. CEPM, we would like to choose a very typical algorithm in the frequent itemset mining domain, the Aprioti algorithm [10], and make a comparison in between.

Based on Apriori we implemented a packing method called ABPM. We used the traces of each day of all the patients and a *min-support* ratio as the input of the Apriori algorithm and the result we get is all the sets with their length ranges from one to the length of the longest sequence of clinical events. *In our case, we set the ratio to 0.08 which is the best ratio we can get considering the running time of the program.* Then we use a simple strategy to pack activities, which goes through the itemsets generated by Apriori from the largest sets to the sets with only one item, and during the traversal every set will be made a package despite those sets which contain any items that has already been included by another package.

Table 2. Evaluation on Simplification degree

	Package number	Largest package	Average package size
ABPM	76	16	1.1
CEPM	65	8	2.0
CEPM-Jr	82	12	1.4

We come up with two aspects for evaluating the packing results, one is the *Simplification degree* and the other is *Accuracy*. *Simplification degree* describes degree of simplifying the scale of different clinical events, which is a good way to evaluate a packing strategy. *Simplification degree* is more objective but it can hardly describe the quality of packages themselves. *Accuracy*, on the other hand, can describe the quality of packages well, but it can be more subjective that the best way so far is asking for the medical practitioners to make evaluations in accordance with the clinical conditions.

As is shown in Table 2, our method 2-level CEPM generates fewer and larger packages than that of ABPM, as the *package number* of CEPM is smaller and the *average package size* almost doubled that of APBM.

To measure the *Accurary* of two algorithms, we ask medical practitioners to help us estimate whether a package is reasonable to carry those activities inside of it, and it turns out that the activities in most of the packages our method CEPM generates are very correlated to each other in practice and medical practitioners can even conclude a topic out of each package, while the items in the packages ABPM generates are kind of random and messy even though some of packages are large in size. We list several representative packages we select from the output of ABPM and CEPM, respectively in Figs. 4(a) and (b). For example, in Fig. 4(b), the activities in the package "Adenosine deaminase" are mostly tests of blood, and "Hepatitis C antibody assay" contains all assays about Hepatitis B and Hepatitis C. However, for the package "Disposable Infusion" shown in Fig. 4(a) which is the largest package that ABPM generates, the items in it range over medicine ("glucose"), test ("determination of urea"), and care ("hospital checkups fee"), which is less accurate and reasonable than the packing result of CEPM.

Based on experiment and evaluation, we demonstrate that compared with Apriori based packing method, our method CEPM is a significant and efficient method which is of more accuracy, stability and tolerance.

5.3 Evaluation on the Two-Level Packing Strategy of CEPM

As is described in detail in Sect. 4.2, in the CEPM algorithm we use a two-level packing strategy that packs clinical events in the category level first and packs on the patient level later.

Here we set up a comparison experiment between CEPM and a simplified version of CEPM called *CEPM-Jr* which skips the category level packing and

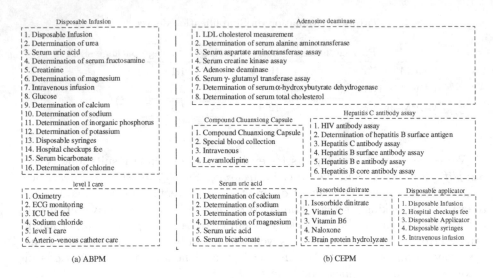

Fig. 4. Package examples from ABPM and CEPM

directly packages clinical events on the patient level. For both algorithm we set the min_sup to 0.8, and the analysis on *Simplification degree* is also shown in Table 2. We can see that CEPM generates fewer and larger packages than CEPM-Jr. As for *Accuracy*, because these two algorithm follows the same strategy, the packages generated by each algorithm are almost all reasonable. Yet CEPM still takes the lead because its packages are more specific than that of CEPM-Jr, as some packages like "LDL cholesterol measurement" in CEPM-Jr packages is sort of divided into two packages in that of CEPM, and considering the fact that under this circumstances the number of CEPM is still smaller than that of CEPM-Jr, it can be indicated that the packing on category level is very effective.

6   Conclusion and Future Work

An innovation of reducing data scale by putting related events into *clinical-event-package*s before an event log is used for process mining and a packing method named CEPM are introduced, and both of them are proved to be able to generate comprehensible and explicable results (both process model and packages) by evaluation of medical practitioners.

Our future work would mainly focus on the following two aspects. One is to enhance the packing method with better packages as output and try to give a proper name to each package. The other is to establish a platform to visualize the packing results as well as process mining results.

Acknowledgments. This work was supported by The National Key Tech- nology R&D Program (No. 2015BAH14F02), and Project 61325008 (Mining and Management of Large Scale Process Data) supported by NSFC.

References

1. Aalst, W., Desel, J., Oberweis, A. (eds.): Business Process Management. LNCS, vol. 1806. Springer, Heidelberg (2000)
2. Günther, C.W., van der Aalst, W.M.P.: Fuzzy mining – adaptive process simplification based on multi-perspective metrics. In: Alonso, G., Dadam, P., Rosemann, M. (eds.) BPM 2007. LNCS, vol. 4714, pp. 328–343. Springer, Heidelberg (2007). doi:10.1007/978-3-540-75183-0_24
3. Lang, M., Bürkle, T., Laumann, S., et al.: Process mining for clinical processes: challenges and current limitations. In: EHealth Beyond the Horizon: Get IT There: Proceedings of MIE2008, the XXIst International Congress of the European Federation for Medical Informatics, p. 229. IOS Press (2008)
4. Gotz, D., Wang, F., Perer, A.: A methodology for interactive mining and visual analysis of clinical event patterns using electronic health record data[J]. J. Biomed. Inform. **48**, 148–159 (2014)
5. Ayres, J., Flannick, J., Gehrke, J., et al.: Sequential pattern mining using a bitmap representation. In: Proceedings of the Eighth ACM SIGKDD International Conference on Knowledge Discovery and Data Mining, pp. 429–435. ACM (2002)
6. Huang, Z., Lu, X., Duan, H.: On mining clinical pathway patterns from medical behaviors. Artif. Intell. Med. **56**(1), 35–50 (2012)
7. Zhang, Y., Padman, R., Wasserman, L.: On learning and visualizing practice-based clinical pathways for chronic kidney disease. In: AMIA Annual Symposium Proceedings, p. 1980. American Medical Informatics Association (2014)
8. Perer, A., Wang, F., Hu, J.: Mining and exploring care pathways from electronic medical records with visual analytics. J. Biomed. Inform. **56**, 369–378 (2015)
9. Günther, C.W., Rozinat, A.: Disco: discover your processes. BPM (Demos) **940**, 40–44 (2012)
10. Agrawal, R., Srikant, R.: Fast algorithms for mining association rules. In: Proceeding 20th International Conference Very Large Data Bases, VLDB, vol. 1215, pp. 487–499 (1994)

A Big Data Analysis Platform for Healthcare on Apache Spark

Jinwei Zhang, Yong Zhang, Qingcheng Hu, Hongliang Tian, and Chunxiao Xing[(✉)]

Tsinghua National Laboratory for Information Science and Technology, Department of Computer Science and Technology, Research Institute of Information Technology, Tsinghua University, Beijing 100084, China
{jinwei-z15,thl12}@mails.tsinghua.edu.cn,
{zhangyong05,huqingcheng,xingcx}@tsinghua.edu.cn

Abstract. In recent years, Data Mining techniques such as classification, clustering, association, regression etc. are widely used in healthcare field to help analyzing and predicting disease and improving the quality and efficiency of medical services. This paper presents a web-based platform for big data analysis of healthcare using Data Mining techniques. The platform consists of three main layers: Apache Spark Layer, Workflow Layer and Web Service Layer. Apache Spark Layer provides basic Apache Spark functionalities as regular Resilient Distributed Datasets (RDD) operations. Meanwhile, this layer provides a cache mechanism to maximize the use of the results as much as possible which were calculated before. Workflow Layer encapsulates a variety of nodes for Data Mining, which have different roles such as data source, algorithm model or evaluation tool. These nodes can be organized into a workflow which is a directed acyclic graph (DAG), and then it will be submitted to Apache Spark Layer to execute. And we have implemented many models including Naïve Bayes model, Decision Tree model and Logistic Regression model etc. for healthcare big data. Web Service Layer implements rich restful API including data uploading, workflow composition and analysis task submission. We also provide a web graphical interface for the user. Through the interface users can achieve efficient Data Mining without any programming which can greatly help the medical staff who don't understand programming to diagnose the patients' condition more accurately and efficiently.

Keywords: Healthcare analysis platform · Cloud computing · Disease prediction · Apache Spark · Big data

This work was supported by the National High-tech R&D Program of China (Grant No. SS2015AA020102), NSFC (91646202), the 1000-Talent program, Tsinghua University Initiative Scientific Research Program.

C. Xing et al. (Eds.): ICSH 2016, LNCS 10219, pp. 32–43, 2017.
DOI: 10.1007/978-3-319-59858-1_4

1 Introduction

In human society, the development of Cloud Computing, Internet of Things and other new services promotes the type and size of data growth at an unprecedented rate. Academia, industry and even government agencies have begun to pay close attention to the big data problems, and more and more people have a strong interest on it. Data Mining is one of the most popular and motivating techniques of discovering meaningful information from varies and huge amount of data. In recent year, Data Mining techniques have been widely used in healthcare field due to its efficient analytical methodology for detecting unknown and valuable information in health data as well as detection of fraud in health insurance, availability of medical solution to the patients at lower cost, detection of causes of diseases and identification of medical treatment methods. It also helps healthcare researchers for making efficient healthcare policies, constructing drug recommendation systems and developing health profiles of individuals [1].

An amount of research works has been done for healthcare using Data Mining techniques. In [2], Data Mining techniques were used to predict Hypertension. And in [3, 4], the authors have utilized classification techniques to predict the likelihood of Cardiovascular Diseases, while in [5, 6], the researchers have put forward integrated Data Mining techniques to detect chronic and physical diseases. Besides, some other researchers [7, 8] developed new methodology and framework for healthcare purpose. However, all of the above-mentioned studies have utilized desktop-based Data Mining techniques. As a result, it's very slow for analyzing the large data.

In the last decade, cloud computing has developed very quickly and provided a new way to establish new healthcare system in a short time with low cost. The "pay for use" pricing model, on-demand computing and ubiquitous network access allow cloud services to be accessible to anyone, anytime, and anywhere [9]. Therefore, it is urgently needed to build an effective big data analysis platform for healthcare which can take advantage of the cloud computing to allow that doctors can quickly and efficiently diagnose the patients' condition. For example, with the help of such platform, doctors can analyze the patient's symptom through the behaviors such as diet, sleep and medical diagnosis history, which will help the doctor gain a more accurate recognition of the patient's condition. Besides, in public health field, the medical big data analysis can also provide healthcare decision-making support, so that patients can get the correct preventive healthcare consulting services and it will change the hospital's medical service model. For medical institutions, the use of big data analysis has become to improve productivity and healthcare services, enhance competitiveness and accelerate economic growth.

Challenges to build such a platform which can handle the large volume of data are as follows:

Challenge I: System Efficiency. As a big data analysis platform, users may not be able to tolerate the long waiting time when handling large data analysis tasks. Therefore, the platform should deal with large data analysis tasks very fast. Besides, for the platform itself, it will take a lot of resources when dealing with the analysis tasks. And of course, we expect that the energy consumption should be meaningful. That is, when a lot of users execute the analysis tasks in the same time period, if the intermediate results are the same among multiple tasks, the platform should be able to reuse these results as much as possible rather than recalculating these tasks from the beginning, which can avoid unnecessary calculation and save the computing resources.

Challenge II: System Scalability. The massive-scale of available multidimensional data hinders using traditional database management systems. Moreover, large-scale multidimensional data, besides its tremendous storage footprint, makes it extremely difficult to manage and maintain. The underlying database system must be able to digest Petabytes of data and effectively analyze it.

Challenge III: User-Friendliness. User may be a professional, but without good programming ability or even if he or she does not understand programming completely. Therefore, it is important to build a visual interface that users who just need very little knowledge of data mining or machine learning can deal with a big data analysis task.

Existing database systems have a whole set of data types, functions, operators and index structures to handle the multidimensional data operations. Even though such systems provide full support for the data storage and access, they suffer from a scalability issue. Based upon a relational database system, such systems are not scalable enough to handle large scale analytics over big data. The Hadoop distributed computing framework based on MapReduce performs data analytics at scale. The Hadoop-based approach indeed achieves high scalability. However, these systems though exhibit excellent performance in batch-processing jobs, they show poor performance in handling applications that require fast data analysis. Apache Spark, on the other hand, is an in-memory cluster computing system. Spark provides a novel data abstraction called resilient distributed datasets (RDDs) that are collections of objects partitioned across a cluster of machines. Each RDD is built using parallelized transformations (filter, join or group by) that could be traced back to recover the RDD data. In-memory RDDs allow Spark to outperform existing models (MapReduce) by up to two orders of magnitude. In fact, this can meet the demand of fast analysis. Unfortunately, when the same job runs on Spark directly twice, both running cost the same time, that is, the Spark takes the same memory and the same CPU time to execute the same job twice, though it can return the results of the last time directly, which causes the waste of resources.

A cloud based framework [10] has been developed for delivering healthcare as a service. In [11], the work provides a Cloud-based adaptive compression and secure management services for 3D healthcare data which mainly focus on dealing with varies kinds of healthcare data types for further disease detection. The work in [12] provides a cloud based framework for home diagnosis over big medical data. All these research works took the advantages of the fast development, scalability, rapid provisioning, instant elasticity, greater resiliency, rapid re-constitution of services, low-cost disaster recovery and data storage solutions made available by cloud computing [13]. However, these systems are not user-friendly and require professional computer sciences engineers to use.

In this paper, we design and implement a big data analysis platform for healthcare which takes advantages of the mature Data Mining techniques in order to produce precise results while at the same time harness the opportunities of advanced distributed computing framework–Apache Spark to offer low cost but high quality services. Our platform significantly lowers the required expertise level for coding and machine learning algorithm with the help of web user interface. In the usual big data analysis research, our system has very good performance for the medical data. Our contributions are as follows:

1. We developed a big data analysis system which can convert user-defined machine learning workflow into an Apache Spark job. The workflow consists of different kinds of nodes that can be data source, preprocessing tool, machine learning model and evaluating tool.
2. We design a cache strategy to use the intermediate results calculated before as much as possible, which makes the analysis faster and hardware resource utilization lower. For every node of the user-defined workflow, we calculate the hash code according to the node's content which includes node inputs and node parameters. When a data analysis job is submitted, the system can use the intermediate results calculated by previous job, if the hash code of the nodes which the intermediate results depend on is the same as the new job's corresponding nodes.
3. Our platform provides a web-based graphical user interface to help users build the big data analysis workflow conveniently and quickly. Users just need very little knowledge of data mining or machine learning, that is, it is enough to deal with a big data analysis task for everyone if the one makes sense of the meaning of every node. Those users who are non-specialized programmer don't need to do any coding and can compose a big data analysis job just by clicking and dragging through the mouse in our website.

We demonstrate our platform using an application: we will create a complex workflow including Decision Tree model, Logistic Regression model and Naïve Bayes model to analyze the medical big data which will show the power of quick analyzing. The effectiveness of the cache strategy is proved by modifying part of the whole workflow.

2   Related Work

This section briefly describes data mining, Apache Spark and LRU cache strategy we used in our work.

2.1   Data Mining

Data Mining is an interdisciplinary subfield of computer sciences [14, 15]. It is the computational process of discovering patterns in large data sets involving methods at the intersection of artificial intelligence, machine learning, statistics, and database systems. The overall goal of the data mining process is to extract information from a data set and transform it into an understandable structure for further use. Data mining is the analysis step of the "knowledge discovery in databases" process.

The actual data mining task is the automatic or semi-automatic analysis of large quantities of data to extract previously unknown, interesting patterns such as groups of data records (cluster analysis), unusual records (anomaly detection), and dependencies (association rule mining). In general, such tasks can be classified into two categories: descriptive and predictive. Descriptive mining tasks include association, clustering, and summarization. These tasks, characterize properties of the data in a target data set. Predictive mining tasks include classification, and regression. They perform induction on the current data in order to make predictions [16].

2.2 Apache Spark

Apache Spark provides programmers with an application programming interface centered on a data structure called the resilient distributed dataset (RDD), a read-only multiset of data items distributed over a cluster of machines, that is maintained in a fault-tolerant way [17]. It was developed in response to limitations in the MapReduce cluster computing paradigm, which forces a particular linear dataflow structure on distributed programs: MapReduce programs read input data from disk, map a function across the data, reduce the results of the map, and store reduction results on disk. Spark's RDDs function as a working set for distributed programs that offers a (deliberately) restricted form of distributed shared memory [18].

Apache Spark can run programs up to 100x faster than Hadoop MapReduce in memory, or 10x faster on disk. Apache Spark has an advanced DAG execution engine that supports cyclic data flow and in-memory computing. Spark powers a stack of libraries including SQL and DataFrames, MLlib for machine learning, GraphX, and Spark Streaming [19].

Spark MLlib is a distributed machine learning framework on top of Spark Core that, due in large part to the distributed memory-based Spark architecture, is as much as nine times as fast as the disk-based implementation used by Apache Mahout and scales better than Vowpal Wabbit. Many common machine learning and statistical algorithms have been implemented and are shipped with MLlib which simplifies large scale machine learning pipelines.

2.3 LRU Cache Strategy

LRU is an abbreviation for Least Recently Used. This cache strategy discards the least recently used items first. And the algorithm requires keeping track of what was used when, which is expensive if one wants to make sure the algorithm always discards the least recently used item. General implementations of this technique require keeping "age bits" for cache-lines and track the "Least Recently Used" cache-line based on age-bits. In such an implementation, every time a cache-line is used, the age of all other cache-lines changes. LRU is actually a family of caching algorithms with members including 2Q by Theodore Johnson and Dennis Shasha [20], and LRU/K by Pat O'Neil, Betty O'Neil and Gerhard Weikum [21].

For CPU caches with large associativity (generally > 4 ways), the implementation cost of LRU becomes prohibitive. In many CPU caches, a scheme that almost always discards one of the least recently used items is sufficient. So many CPU designers choose a PLRU algorithm which only needs one bit per cache item to work. PLRU typically has a slightly worse miss ratio, has a slightly better latency, uses slightly less power than LRU and lower overheads compared to LRU.

3   Platform Architecture

As depicted in Fig. 1, our platform consists of three main layers: (1) Apache Spark Layer (Sect. 3.1). (2) Workflow Layer (Sect. 3.2). (3) Web Service Layer (Sect. 3.3).

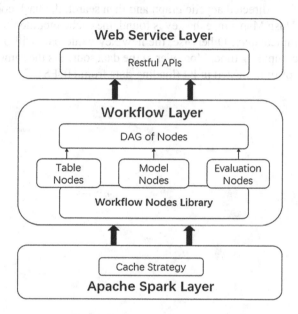

Fig. 1. The architecture of the platform

3.1   Apache Spark Layer

This layer consists of regular operations that are natively supported by Apache Spark and responsible for loading/saving data from/to persistent storage which is either local disk or Hadoop file system HDFS according to the file type and other RDD operations of transformation and action to execute some user-defined workflow. Besides, we design a cache strategy in this layer.

Storage Strategy. For the multidimensional big data needed to analyze, we will generate a scheme file which describe the data type for every column. The DataFrame is a distributed collection of data organized into named columns. It is conceptually equivalent to a table in a relational database or a data frame in R/Python, but with richer optimizations under the hood. When we generate a DataFrame object from the multi-dimensional big data, we need the corresponding scheme file. Because the scheme file size is very small about a few KB and the HDFS block size is 64 MB at least, so we store the scheme file on the local file system and the data on HDFS.

Cache Strategy. Figure 2 displays a workflow for medical data analysis. Users can click the node of the workflow to view the data or the configuration of the node. We will cache every output of the node and put the intermediate results into a Hash Map. And the key corresponding to the intermediate result is a string of hash code which is calculated according to the input and parameters of the node that is the data and configuration of the node. When the user-defined workflow is executed on the Apache Spark layer, the system will firstly call the cache strategy module to calculate every node's hash code from the origin of the directed acyclic graph and then search the hash code string from the key set of the Hash Map. Once the key is found, the cache module returns the corresponding value immediately. Otherwise, the new key-value pair will be cached. This will save a lot of computing time. Moreover, if the data source is the same as the before, we can save a lot of time wasted in IO (loading data from HDFS).

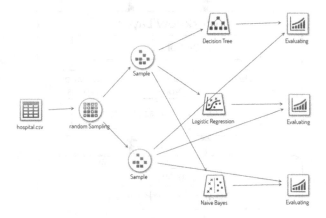

Fig. 2. An example work flow

But memory is limited and the Hash Map will certainly not increase without limit. So we designed an evict policy based LRU algorithm for key-value pairs of the Hash Map. We set the maximum number for key-value pairs in the Hash Map and let a positive integer to indicate the key-value pair's access time. "1" indicates that the key-value pair is accessed just now or a new item. The bigger the integer is; the easier the corresponding key-value pair is evicted from the Map.

On Apache Spark, analysis task of multi-submission using the cache data depends on that they share one Spark Context, that is, there are many jobs belonging to one Spark Application. We set the whole web service as the Spark Application to ensure this. Because the web listening service is a daemon process, the Spark Context will always exist after an analysis task has finished.

3.2 Work Flow Layer

This layer encapsulates a variety of nodes of machine learning workflow, for example, table node that is regard as the data source, model nodes are machine learning algorithm models including decision tree node, logistic regression node and so on, evaluation nodes are used to evaluate the results calculated by the model nodes. Besides, it converts the user-defined workflow to a directed acyclic graph and identifies the validity of the DAG. The validation involves two aspects: on the one hand we will verify whether if the workflow is really a DAG, on the other hand we will verify whether if the DAG is legal, that is, whether the nodes meet the correlation between each other. For example, the table node is the data source, so it must be the origin of some DAG and the DAG must be illegal if there is any node as the prefix of the table node.

In fact, we develop a library named workflowLib to allow programmers to develop all kinds of workflow nodes more conveniently. There are mainly two abstract classes in the library: JobNode class and JobNodeParam class. And there is an abstract function named computeResult in the JobNode class. The abstract function needs to define the detail operations for the node, which defines how to deal with the input and get the output. If the programmers want to add a new machine learning model, he or she just needs to define a class which inherits the JobNode class and implement the abstract function computeResult. Accordingly, the programmer needs to implement the JobNodeParam class to define the parameters for the node. The developers don't need to care about how to verify the DAG. They just need to add the new node defined to a workflow.

The user-defined workflow is a JSON file as the input of this layer. According to the detailed definition of every node of the workflow, the workflow layer module will generate a DAG and then submit it to the Apache Spark Layer.

3.3 Web Service Layer

This layer provides the web service to users, which has two functions. On the one hand, users can deal with big data analysis task on our platform without developing the algorithm themselves. For example, they just need to send a JSON file over HTTP request, which will create a workflow on our platform. On the other hand, the whole platform is really a web service running on the Apache Spark as a daemon process that is a Spark Application which guarantees that the Spark Context always exists. This is the base of the cache strategy described in Sect. 2.1.

The web service layer provides rich Restful APIs including upload the data, delete the data, create a workflow, modify a workflow, execute a workflow and so on.

4 Experiment

In this session, we will display our platform using an analytical application which is described below. The data set used in the display is the medical data, which has almost 45000 items and 43 dimensions. We provide a web user interface to be convenient for users to analyze. A screenshot of this tool's main interface "Workflows" is provided in Fig. 3. The tool has a shockingly simple user interface, so that no programming technical background is needed and you just do your analysis for big data using just drag and drop with the mouse. Figure 3 displays a new blank workflow, where you can customize your own analyzing workflow. On the left side of Fig. 3, there are nodes that are used to create the workflow. The menu of "Tables" in Fig. 3 shows data resources that are uploaded by users through the upload function in "Tables" interface. The menu of "Preparation" in Fig. 3 includes Random Sampling node, Sample node, Filter node, Join node and Select node which are used to preprocess the data source. There are some machine learning algorithm models including Decision Tree node, Logistic Regression node, Naïve Bayes node, Linear Regression node, Gradient Boosting node, K-Means node and Support Vector Machine node in "Models" menu. In the "Evaluating" menu, there are Scoring node and Evaluating node which are used to identify the training model. Figure 4 shows the "Tables Management" interface which provides functions including uploading file, creating folder, deleting file or folder and moving the file, etc. Because there were some projects using our platform, you can see some tables listed in Fig. 4. All uploading files through the uploading function in Fig. 4 will be listed in the "Tables" menu in Fig. 3. User can just drag and drop the nodes listed on the left side of "Work-flows" interface into the middle section of Fig. 3. When you drag a node into the work-flow, the system will help you combine the dragging node with nodes that have been in the workflow automatically, if one's output can be the input of the other.

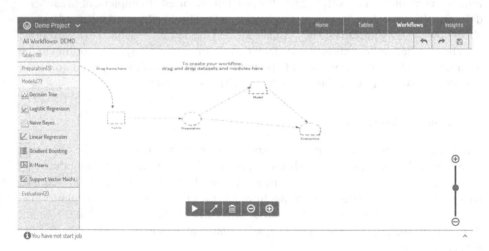

Fig. 3. The main interface of our platform

We will use the workflow displayed in Fig. 2 to demonstrate the big data analyzing. When a user clicks the "Run button" that is a triangle in Fig. 3, all of the nodes will be gray and if one node's job has been finished, the node will be lighted up. There is an upward arrow in the bottom right corner of Fig. 3 and a user can look over the log information by clicking that arrow. Users can click any node to configure it. For example, the Random Sampling node can define the percent of training set and testing set and the Decision Tree node can configure the training target from the 43 dimensions in the data set and it can also define the parameters for the process of constructing the Decision

Tree which is displayed in Fig. 5. When all of the nodes have lighted up, the whole workflow is completed. Users can click the "Evaluating" nodes to view the results for the big data analysis.

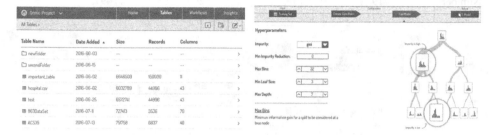

Fig. 4. The data sources   **Fig. 5.** The result

Because the results of every time for random sampling are different, the input of nodes of the same workflow is different except the table node. In order to present our cache strategy, we divide the table node into two parts manually, and execute the same workflow twice. But there is a little of difference that we change the target of the Decision Tree node. In the first execution, the running time of the Logistic Regression node is more than the Decision Tree node's obviously. But the opposite occurs in the second execution. Because the input and configuration are the same in two executions for the Logistic Regression node, the results of it should be same. Indeed, that is also the fact, which indicates our cache strategy is correct and effective.

We know that it's the presupposition and key to analyze the hospital's electronic medical records data(EMR) for the Clinical Decision Support System. In this paper, we will take the acute chest pain data analysis process as an example to display the excellence of our platform.

Firstly, we selected 1571 data items of cardiovascular patients from the acute chest pain information database, which includes four kinds of cardiovascular disease, that is, aortic dissection, pulmonary embolism, myocardial infarction and steno cardia. The detail information of the data is displayed in Table 1. We extract 31 disease features from patients' symptoms and signs, history feature, laboratory inspection and so on. And then, we pre-processed the data of qualitative variables and quantitative variables in 31 pathologic features and according to the actual data characteristics we get the final 17 pathologic features to analyze. Finally, we take advantage of the Decision Tree model, Naïve Bayes model and Logistic Regression model to predict the incidence of the four kinds of cardiovascular disease. Figure 6 displays the weights influence of each disease feature on different diseases using Logistic Regression model. And Fig. 7 displays the prediction accuracy of Logistic Regression model. From Fig. 7, we can find that the prediction accuracy for aortic dissection is more than 99%, but just 64% for pulmonary embolism, which is because the amount of data for pulmonary embolism is relatively small and only 78/1571 of the total data.

Table 1. Data of cardiovascular patients.

Disease	Aortic dissection	Pulmonary embolism	Myocardial infarction	Steno cardia
Number	719	78	266	497
Total	1571			

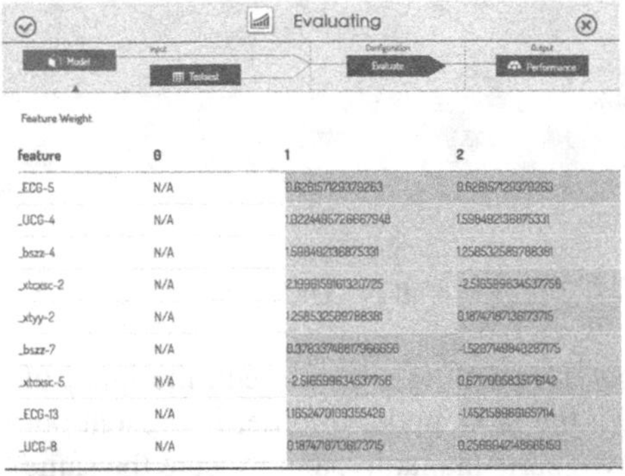

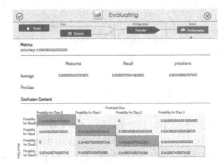

Fig. 6. The weights influence of each disease feature

Fig. 7. prediction accuracy of LR model

5   Conclusion

We develop a web service platform on Apache Spark for big data analysis on healthcare data. In our system, we propose a cache strategy to realize the high efficiency of the system, which does not exist in other big data analyzing platform as we know. And in Workflow Layer, we develop a workflowLib which indeed is a framework for implementing user-defined nodes of workflow of machine learning. Besides, we develop a web user interface through which anyone can do the big data analyzing easily. At present, there are some big data analysis tasks running on our platform and it presents a good performance.

In the future, we will develop a stronger platform on which users can write own code for the model nodes in the web user interface when the nodes we provide cannot meet their demands. We will also compile the user-writing code to a model node that will be provided to others directly if the user agrees to publish the code.

References

1. Koh, H.C., Tan, G.: Data mining application in healthcare. J. Healthcare Inf. Manage. **19**(2) (2005)
2. Aljumah, A.A., Ahamad, M.G., Siddiqui, M.K.: Predictive analysis on hypertension treatment using data mining approach in Saudi Arabia. Intell. Inf. Manage. **3**, 252–261 (2011)
3. Dangare, C.S., Apte, S.S.: Improved study of heart disease prediction system using data mining classification techniques (2012)

4. Kumari, M., Godara, S.: Comparative study of data mining classification methods in cardiovascular disease prediction. IJCST **2**(2) (2011). ISSN: 2229- 4333
5. Huang, M.-J., Chen, M.-Y., Lee, S.-C.: Integrating data mining with case-based reasoning for chronic diseases prognosis and diagnosis. Expert Syst. Appl. **32**, 856–867 (2007)
6. Ha, S.H., Joo, S.H.: A hybrid data mining method for the medical classification of chest pain. Int. J. Comput. Inf. Eng. **4**(1), 33–38 (2010)
7. Amendola, S., Lodato, R., Manzari, S., et al.: RFID technology for IoTbased personal healthcare in smart spaces. IEEE Internet Things J. **1**(2), 144–152 (2014)
8. Jung, E.Y., Kim, J., Chung, K.Y., et al.: Mobile healthcare application with EMR interoperability for diabetes patients. Cluster Comput. **17**(3), 871–880 (2014)
9. Armbrust, M., Fox, A., Griffith, R., Joseph, A.D., Katz, R.H., Konwinski, A., Lee, G., Patterson, D.A., Rabkin, A., Stoica, I., Zaharia, M.: Above the Clouds: A Berkeley View of Cloud Computing, UCB/EECS 2009-28, 10 February 2009
10. Kaur, P.D., Chana, I.: Cloud based intelligent system for delivering healthcare as a service. Comput. Methods Programs Biomed. **113**(1), 346–359 (2014)
11. Castiglione, A., Pizzolante, R., De Santis, A., et al.: Cloud-based adaptive compression and secure management services for 3D healthcare data. Future Gener. Comput. Syst. **43**, 120–134 (2015)
12. Lin, W., Dou, W., Zhou, Z., et al.: A cloud-based framework for Home diagnosis service over big medical data. J. Syst. Softw. **102**, 192–206 (2015)
13. Buyya, R., Yeo, C.S., Venugopal, S., Broberg, J., Brandic, I.: Cloud computing and emerging IT platforms: vision hype, and reality for delivering computing as the 5th utility. Future Gener. Comput. Syst. **25**(6), 599–616 (2009)
14. Clifton, C.: Encyclopædia Britannica: Definition of Data Mining (2010). Accessed 09 Dec 2010
15. Hastie, T., Tibshirani, R., Friedman, J.: The Elements of Statistical Learning: Data Mining, Inference, and Prediction. Accessed 07 Aug 2012
16. Wolford, D.K.: System, pad and method for monitoring a sleeping person to detect an apnea state condition: U.S, Patent Application 12/359,459[P] (2009)
17. Zaharia, M., Chowdhury, M., Franklin, M.J., Shenker, S., Stoica, I.: Spark: cluster computing with working sets (PDF). In: USENIX Workshop on Hot Topics in Cloud Computing (HotCloud)
18. Zaharia, M., Chowdhury, M., Das, T., Dave, A., Ma, J., McCauley, M., Franklin, M.J., Shenker, S., Stoica, I.: Resilient distributed datasets: a fault-tolerant abstraction for in-memory cluster computing (PDF). In: USENIX Symposium Networked Systems Design and Implementation
19. Sparks, E., Talwalkar, A.: Spark Meetup: MLbase, distributed machine learning with spark. In: slideshare.net. Spark User Meetup, San Francisco, California (2013). slideshare.net, Accessed 10 Feb 2014
20. Johnson, T., Dennis, S.: X3: A Low Overhead High Performance Buffer Management Replacement Algorithm (1994)
21. O'neil, E.J., O'neil, P.E., Weikum, G.: The LRU-K page replacement algorithm for database disk buffering. In: Proceedings of the 1993 ACM SIGMOD International Conference on Management of Data. SIGMOD 1993, pp. 297–306. ACM, New York (1993)

A Semi-automated Entity Relation Extraction Mechanism with Weakly Supervised Learning for Chinese Medical Webpages

Zhao Liu[1,2], Jian Tong[1,2], Jinguang Gu[1,2(✉)], Kai Liu[1,2], and Bo Hu[3]

[1] College of Computer Science and Technology,
Wuhan University of Science and Technology, Wuhan 430065, China
simongu@qq.com
[2] Hubei Province Key Laboratory of Intelligent Information Processing
and Real-Time Industrial System, Wuhan 430065, China
[3] Kingdee Cloud Platform Department,
Kingdee International Software Group Co., Ltd., Shenzhen 518057, China

Abstract. Medical entity relation extraction is of great significance for medical text data mining and medical knowledge graph. However, medical field requires very high data accuracy rate, the current medical entity relation extraction system is difficult to achieve the required accuracy. A main technical difficulty lies in how to obtain high-precision medical data, and automatically generate annotated training sample set. In this paper, a medical entity relation automatic extraction system based on weak supervision is proposed. At first, we designed a visual annotation tool, it can automatically generate crawl scripts, crawling the medical data from the site where the entity and its attributes are Separate stored. Then, based on the acquired data structure, we propose a weakly supervised hypothesis to automatically generate positive sample training data. Finally, we use CNN model to extract medical entity relation. Experiments show that the method is feasible and accurate.

Keywords: Medical entity · Entity relation extraction · Convolutional neural network · Weakly supervised learning

1 Introduction

With the rapid development of the Internet, people are increasingly inclined to find medical information online. According to Baidu's latest official statistics, medical-related information is searched more than 170 million times per day. 2015 Baidu and the China Association for Science and Technology released the "Chinese Internet users popular science demand search behavior report" based on the Baidu Index. Report shows that "Health and medical" has become the most concerned science theme for Internet users, Ratio as high as 57%. This shows that users of medical information online access has a great demand. But people often need to browse a lot of irrelevant information in order to obtain the information of interest. The construction of Chinese medical knowledge graph can solve this problem. Knowledge graph provide the ability to analyze problems from a "relation" perspective, Users can

© Springer International Publishing AG 2017
C. Xing et al. (Eds.): ICSH 2016, LNCS 10219, pp. 44–56, 2017.
DOI: 10.1007/978-3-319-59858-1_5

quickly and effectively access the relevant knowledge and the logical relation between knowledge. For example, users search for hypertension, the system should be able to accurately display the information such as cause, related symptoms, treatment and complications. We can see that the relation extraction [1] is an important part.

Currently the main method of relation extraction can be divided into three categories: pattern matching, dictionary-driven and machine learning. Although the first two methods have high accuracy, but they need experts to manually develop rules, time-consuming and poor portability. While the machine learning method in the case of sufficient training data, can also achieve a high accuracy, so machine learning methods are increasingly receiving attention. Traditional machine learning methods such as SVM, Naive Bayesian and k-neighbor algorithm has been extensively applied to relational extraction researches. But the machine learning method needs a lot of training corpus. The adequacy of corpus plays a vital role in the quality of training results. How to automatically generate a large number of accurate training corpus by using the existing knowledge base without manual annotation is a difficult problem.

This paper presents an automated solution, we captured the relation between entity and attributes in medical websites, the weakly supervised training method was used to generate the positive sample training set, and the entity relation was extracted by convolution neural network model. The core technical difficulty lies in how to extract entity and its attribute description data from the medical websites which stores entities separated from their attributes, and how to use the weakly supervised method to generate the positive sample training corpus by using the captured medical data.

Medical websites contain a wealth of entity and attribute description data, but the entities and their attributes in medical web sites tend to be distributed in different pages [16]. So this paper puts forward a kind of automation extraction system for the structure of the entity attributes separated storage. This system not only can complete separate storage entity and attribute extraction, but also compatible with the conventional extraction of the single page level. Can be used as a preliminary medical data collection and processing platform

After obtaining the entity attribute description data, we need to generate the entity description at sentence level at first, and then use the weakly supervised method to generate the positive sample training data which contains the entity and its attribute relation. Finally, we use the convolution neural network to extract the relation. How to use weak supervision method to generate positive sample training data is also a highlight of this paper. Convolution neural network is a kind of effective recognition method which has been developed recently years and has attracted wide attention. As a kind of classification model, convolution neural network can also have a very good deal with relation extraction problem. Therefore this paper uses the convolution neural network model as a classifier to identify the relation of medical entities.

The rest of this paper is organized as follows: Sect. 2 introduces the related work in the field of entity relation extraction. In Sect. 3, the relation extraction method of this paper is introduced in detail. And Sect. 4 is the experiment and result analysis. The last section is the discussion and conclusion.

2 Related Work

Relation extraction is one of the tasks of information extraction, can be divided into binary relation extraction and multiple relation extraction. In recent years, there are many kinds of entity extraction methods, most of them are machine learning based on supervised learning methods or weakly supervised learning methods. Supervised learning methods can be divided into two methods: feature vector based method and kernel function based method. Eigenvector-based methods focus on the extraction of discriminative features to describe local features or entity features in relational instances. The method in [2] considers the entities, the entity types, the dependency tree and the parse tree, and then uses the maximum entropy classifier to judge the relations among the entities. Zhou et al. [3] systematically studied how to combine various features, including basic phrase blocks, and discussed the contribution of various linguistic features to relational extraction performance. Jiang et al. [4] studied the influence of different features on the relation extraction performance through a uniform feature space expression. The feature space can be divided into feature subspace, such as sequence, syntax tree and dependency tree. Although the method based on eigenvector is very fast and effective, its disadvantage is that a feature set needs to be explicitly given when transforming structured features. Because of the complexity and variability of semantic relations among entities, it is difficult to further improve the performance of relational extraction, because it is difficult to find new effective vocabulary, syntactic or semantic features suitable for semantic relation extraction. Different from eigenvector method, the method based on kernel function is to deal with the tree directly. When calculating the distance between the relations, the kernel function is used to implicitly calculate the distance between objects in the high-dimensional feature space. Instead of enumerating all the features, it is possible to calculate the dot product of the vector, indicating that the entity relation is more flexible. Zelenk et al. [5] proposed Kernel-based relational extraction firstly, and they defined the tree kernel function on the basis of the shallow syntax tree of the text and designed a dynamic programming algorithm of the similarity of the calculation tree kernel function, then, the semantic relations among entities are extracted by support vector machine (SVM) and voting algorithm (VotedPerceptron). Zhang et al. [6] considered the planar and structural features that affect the semantic relations among entities, The similarity between the syntactic trees containing entity pairs is calculated by using the convolution tree kernel function, and the similarity between the entity attributes (such as the entity type) is calculated using the linear kernel function. Zhou et al. [7] proposed that the shortest path contains the tree core, and the semantic relation instance is represented as the context-dependent shortest path inclusion tree. The kernel function is combined with the feature-based approach.

Relation extraction based on weakly supervised learning is first put forward by literature [8], used for abstracting the relation between proteins and genes from abstracts of academic literature. In [9], weak-supervised relation extraction is regarded as a multi-example problem. [10] not only model the noise training data, and model the entity that may belong to multiple relation types. In the literature [11], the pseudo relevance feedback in information retrieval is used to overcome the problem of sample noise. In [12], the density of the sample space is used to obtain the spatial geometric features of the response data. On the basis of this, they use the mark transfer method to make the similar vertexes, give the same class mark as possible, and use a large number of unknown pattern samples for weak supervised learning at last.

Convolutional neural network is a kind of artificial neural network, which is used in the field of image recognition. When the image and the text are directly used as the input of the network, the convolutional neural network can construct a large number of redundant features directly from the original data, which can reduce the complex feature extraction and data reconstruction process. So in recent years, the convolutional neural network is effectively used in various field of natural language processing tasks, including: In recent years, convolution neural networks have also been applied to a variety of natural language processing tasks, including: part of speech tagging, noun phrase recognition, named entity recognition, semantic role labeling [13], semantic analysis [14], sentence model And classification [15], relation classification and extraction.

3   Automation Medical Entity Relation Extraction System Based on Weakly Supervised Learning

In this paper, the relation extraction process is divided into two parts. The first step is to obtain medical data from the major medical websites. In order to facilitate the training system behind, the data here is contains medical entity and its attributes. The final results format is shown in Table 1. The second step is to extract the relation between the medical entities in the medical data. The complete flow of the experiment is shown in Fig. 1.

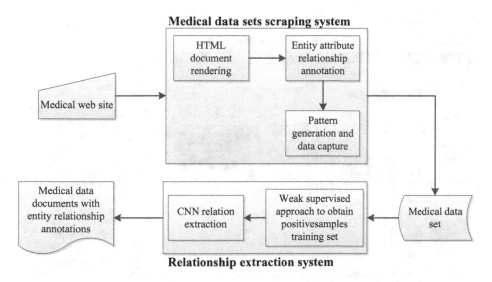

Fig. 1. Medical entity relation based on weakly supervised learning

3.1 Medical Entity and Attribute Data Fetching

Medical Web site is an important research data resource of medical information technology research and development. But the observation found that most of the medical data are embedded in the template or script to dynamically generate the pages. And the characteristic of medical data storage is that an entity and its attributes are often distributed in different page. The current crawling system focuses on website which entity and its attributes stored in a single web page, cannot effectively complete the crawl task. So this paper puts forward a kind of automation extraction system for the structure of the entity attributes separated storage. The system is divided into three steps to complete data collection.

HTML Document Rendering. This interface consists of two modules, as shown in Fig. 2. (As the copyright issues, Wanfang database cannot be made public. So here is an another medical website as example) On the left is a container for the page to be labeled, and the right part is used as an action option for the user to mark the page. In the system address bar to enter the page URL, click the "Show page" button, system will get HTML documents by the HTTP protocol, and display web pages in the container on the left side of the system. At the same time it use the browser rendering engine to parse HTML documents and build a DOM tree. User can click page combined with control on the right to operate.

Entity Attribute Relation Annotation. When the entity and its corresponding attribute exists in the same page, the user only need to mark the entity and attribute relations in the single page, and when the relation between entities and attributes distributed in different web pages, the annotation module can help users access to the target property page and record user actions, by remembering the relation between them to infer the relation between data.

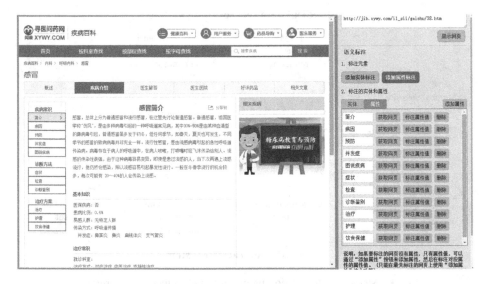

Fig. 2. Extraction system interface

Algorithm 1 Annotation Algorithm

```
Begin
1: Function GetSelectorPath()
2: if e is root element then
3:    return p
4: end if
5: t = e.name
6: s = e.cssSelector()
7: p = t + s
8: return p + GetSelectorPath(e.parent)
End
```

Entity annotation refers to the user needs to label entities and its attribute description information. Web page annotation algorithm based on JavaScript and CSS selector technology, As shown in Algorithm 1. Algorithm 1 locates the position of the current label element by acquiring the position of the mouse, and use the CSS selector chain to represent the location of the dimension element. For example, when a user uses the mouse to label an entity (DOM structure shown in Fig. 3), we get the position of the entity in the page at first, and then we get the CSS selector path to the entity. The resulting CSS selector path will be inserted into the corresponding DOM tree property "data-selector"(custom property), and be used to generate decimation patterns.

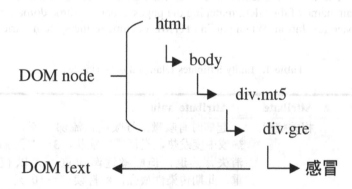

Fig. 3. DOM structure of the cold entity

Pattern Generation and Data Extraction. In this step, we generate the extraction pattern by using the information that the user has annotated. The CSS selector path corresponding to the entity and attribute relations that have been marked will be logged, and Then generate nested grab rules for data extraction. The system uses JSON format to store the crawled data information.

Algorithm 2 shows the process of converting annotation information into extraction pattern. The algorithm receives the user-annotated entity and all the corresponding attribute descriptions. Entity and attribute are part of the DOM structure tree, and carry the corresponding CSS selector path and the address information of the web page.

Algorithm 2 generates extraction pattern

```
begin
 1: Function ConstructPattern(entity,attribute)
 2: pattern = {}, and attr = {}
 3: pattern.entitySelector = entity.path
 4: #attribute = number(attribute)
 5: foreach i in (0,#attribute) then
 6:    attr.url = url of attributes
 7:    attr.nameSelector = path of attribute
 8:    attr.valSelector = value path of attribute
 9:    pattern.push(attr)
10: end for
11: return pattern
end
```

After extracting pattern generation, you can use it for data extraction. This system uses breadth-first algorithm search page website, then use the generated nested pattern to match the page HTML document, get data matching relation between the entity and its attributes. The whole extraction process is: First get the URL of the annotated page, get the domain name of the URL, matching the pages under the same domain name one by one for page resolution; When parsing HTML document, the system retrieves all of

Table 1. Entity attributes relational data samples

Entity	Attribute	Attribute value
	相关症状	起病时有咳嗽，打喷嚏，流涕，流泪，有低热或中度发热，类似感冒症状，3～4 天后症状消失，热退，但咳嗽逐渐加重，尤以夜间为重，此期传染性最强，可持续 7～10 天，若及时治疗，能有效地控制本病的发展。因缺氧而出现发钳，甚至于抽搐，亦可因窒息而死亡。
百日咳	相关检查	1、血液检查：在卡他期末及痉咳早期白细胞计数高达(20～40)×109/L，最高可达 100×109/L，分类淋巴细胞在 60%以上，亦有高达 90%以上者。2、细菌培养：目前认为鼻咽拭培养法优于咳碟法
	……	……

the URLs in the document for page searches, and then uses the generated pattern to match the HTML document; If the CSS selector path in the nested rule matches a branch path in the document tree, the data record corresponding to the path is fetched and the extracted result is obtained. The finally resulting data is shown in Table 1.

3.2 Using Convolution Neural Network for Relation Extraction

Through the previous step of the crawl, the entity and its attribute description data can be obtained, in which the entity attribute value is unstructured text, and the entity has a certain relation with the medical entity contained in the attribute value text. In this paper, a weakly supervised approach is used to generate a positive training set based on reasonable assumptions and rule constraints. The training data structure is shown in Fig. 5. Convolutional Neural Networks (CNN) model is used to extract relational data.

Weakly Supervised Relation Extraction of the Training Sample. Machine learning requires a large amount of positive sample training data. The manual labeling method requires professional domain knowledge and consumes a large amount of time. A practical and effective relation extraction method should reduce the time consuming and poor consistency of artificial label data, and automatically acquire the positive sample training data. The main idea of the weakly supervised sample extraction is how to automatically generate training samples of positive samples, mainly based on the weakly supervised hypothesis: if the two entities have relations in the knowledge base, it can be inferred that the statements containing the two entities also have the relation in the knowledge base. Although the extracted sample of the weakly supervised relation can automatically generate the training corpus, it also has the problem of carrying noise. As shown in Fig. 4, the first statement expresses the entity-to-relation '并发症'. However, the second statement cannot express this relation. The wrong sample is the back-labeled noise. This noise generation is due to the weak supervisory assumption that there is too little constraint on the generated sample data.

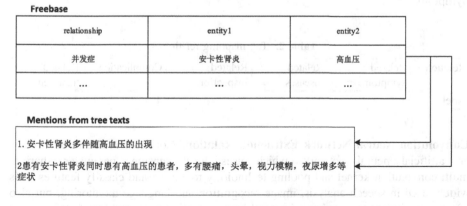

Fig. 4. Example of a weak supervisor relation extraction data generation process

According to the particularity of the data structure. We propose such a weak supervision hypothesis: attribute value is a descriptive text for an entity attribute, generally contain entity of relation to the original entity.

And the training data generation script has the following constraints:

1. The original entity itself acts as the beginning of the sentence in the callback statement and acts as the first entity in the relation.
2. Identify another medical entity in the corresponding attribute value according to the entity attribute.
3. For attribute values, when a sentence contains multiple medical entities, only the first identified entity is used as the entity pair.

Finally we can get the statement (training corpus) as shown in Fig. 5:

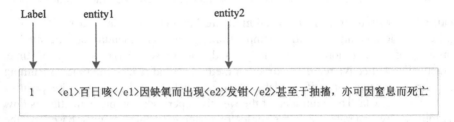

Fig. 5. Training corpus example

- 1: the label (label correspondence shown in Table 2)
- <e1>百日咳</e1>: whooping cough, indicating the entity 1 to be labeled
- <e2>发钳</e2>: cyanosis, indicating the entity 2 to be labeled

The meaning of this statement is that the relation between the entity "pertussis" and the entity "cyanosis" is labeled "1", that is, the entity-to-pair relation as Related Symptoms.

Table 2. Tag mapping relation

Relation	Related symptoms	Related diseases	Related inspection	Complication	Related treatment
label	1	2	3	4	5

Convolution Neural Network Extraction Relation. Convolution neural network is an artificial neural network, which uses local sensing, parameter sharing, multi-convolution kernel and pooling technology to extract and classify features. It is widely used in speech analysis, image recognition and language monitoring, but also effectively applied to a variety of natural language processing problems.

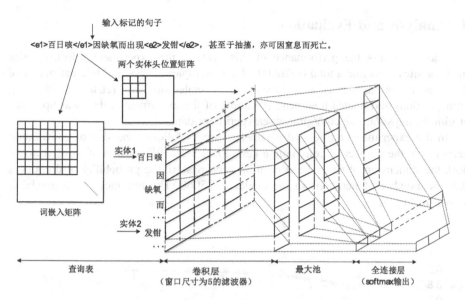

Fig. 6. Structure of relation extraction based on convolutional neural network

As shown in Fig. 6, the convolutional neural network used in this experiment includes the Convolution Max Pooling and the softmax classification.

Convolution neural network input must be in the form of matrix, so the first sentence to be input into the word vector, word vector expression in two ways, one is One-hot expression, the other is the Distributed expression. One-hot expression is the use of high-dimensional vector to represent each word, the vector dimension is the size of the vocabulary, the vector component is only one value is 1, where the vast majority of elements to 0,1 on behalf of the current position of the word. This representation is susceptible to the dimensionality catastrophe, and there is a "word gap" (any two words are isolated) phenomenon. The basic idea of the Distributed expression method is to represent a word directly with a low-dimensional real vector. It can capture the semantic information between words by calculating the distance between the word and the word.

In this paper, it use the word2vec toolkit to transform the training data into the word vector form and obtain the vector matrix. In order to record the position information of the entity, the entity position matrix is obtained by taking the head position of the entity as the position coordinate of the entity. The word vector matrix and the position matrix are merged into the input matrix X of the model.

The matrix is input to the convolution layer for automatic extraction of higher level features. For the pooled layer, there are N input maps and N output maps, but each input map's dimensions are smaller, because it only retains the effective information to obtain the final salient features. The classification operation is the last operation of the convolutional neural network. First, dropout is used to normalize the operation. Dropout In the process of training the network, you can randomly remove some neurons, keep input and output layers unchanged, in this way to prevent over-fitting problem. Then the features of the dropout process are categorized by the softmax classifier model.

4   Analysis and Evaluation

In order to assess the performance of this system, the experiment selected seven medical sites, generate a total of 20000 labeled samples at last, and five categories of directional relations are set: Related symptoms, related diseases, related examination, complications and related treatment. A sample of the experimental data was uploaded at github: https://github.com/gitbrowse/experiment-data.

In the experiment, the related parameters are as follows: the size of convolution kernel is 5, the number of convolution kernel is 150, the dimension of word vector is 300, the dimension of entity head position vector is 10, the probability of dropout is 0.5, the number of iterations of the model is 25000. The accuracy of the model is shown in Fig. 7.

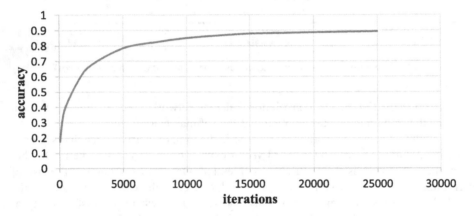

Fig. 7. CNN model training accuracy curve

The experiment is compared with traditional machine learning classification methods: Decision Tree, k-Nearest Neighbors, Gaussian Naive Bayes and SVM. The results are shown in Table 3.

Table 3. The performance evaluation of the method and the traditional machine learning method

Algorithm	Accuracy	Recall rate	F1-Score
Our Method	91.87%	91.58%	0.8908
SVM	83.24%	81.49%	0.7768
Decision Tree	75.33%	75.62%	0.7546
K-nearest Neighbors	79.61%	79.45%	0.7864
Gaussian Naive Bayes	76.19%	71.47%	0.7258
Random Forest	81.54%	81.73%	0.8067

It can be seen from the data in Table that the method of convolutional neural network in this paper is about 10% higher in accuracy, recall rate and F1-Score performance evaluation than the traditional machine learning classification method.

5 Conclusion

In this paper, the data of the entity and its attributes are extracted from the medical web site, as the original corpus of the training. An automatic extraction system for entity attribute separation storage is proposed, which is used to obtain the entities and its attributes. According to the attribute description data of the entity, the entity description of the sentence level is generated, and the sample extraction scheme based on the weak supervisor relation extraction is proposed to find the positive sample training data which contains the entity and its attribute relation. The results are compared with other machine learning methods, and the validity and accuracy of the weakly supervised relation extraction based on convolutional neural network are verified by experiments.

Acknowledgement. This work is supported by the National Natural Science Foundation of China (61272110, 61602350), the Key Projects of National Social Science Foundation of China (11&ZD189), the State Key Lab of Software Engineering Open Foundation of Wuhan University (SKLSE2012-09-07) and NSF of Wuhan University of Science and technology Of China under grant number 2016xz016.

References

1. Sarawagi, S.: Information extraction. J. Found. Trends Databases **3**(1), 261–377 (2008)
2. Kambhatl, N.A.: Combining lexical, syntactic, and semantic features with maximum entropy models for extracting relations. In: The 42nd Annual Meeting on Association for Computational Linguistics on Interactive Poster and Demonstration Sessions, Association for Computational Linguistics, Stroudsburg (2004)
3. Zhou, G.D., Su, J., Zhang, J., Zhang, M.: Exploring various knowledge in relation extraction. In: The 43rd Annual Meeting on Association for Computational Linguistics, pp, 427–434. Association for Computational Linguistics, Stroudsburg (2005)
4. Jiang, J., Zhai, C.X.: A systematic exploration of the feature space for relation extraction. In: Proceedings of Human Language Technologies 2007 and the North American Chapter of the Association for Computational Linguistics, pp. 113–120. Association for Computational Linguistics, Stroudsburg (2007)
5. Zelenko, D., Aone, C., Richardella, A.: Kernel methods for relation extraction. J. Mach. Learn. Res. **3**, 1083–1106 (2003)
6. Zhang, M., Zhang, J., Su, J., Zhou, G.D.: A composite kernel to extract relations between entities with both flat and structured features. In: The 21st International Conference on Computational Linguistics and the 44th Annual Meeting of the Association for Computational Linguistics, pp. 825–832. Association for Computational Linguistics, Stroudsburg (2006)

7. Zhou, G.D., Zhang, M., Ji, D.H., Zhu, Q.M.: Tree kernel-based relation extraction with context-sensitive structured parse tree information. In: The 2007 Joint Conference on Empirical Methods in Natural Language Processing and Computational Natural Language Learning, pp. 728–736 (2007)
8. Craven M., Kumlien J.: Constructing biological knowledge bases by extracting information from text sources. In: The 7th International Conference on Intelligent Systems for Molecular Biology, pp. 77–86. AAAI, Heidelberg(1999)
9. Riedel, S., Yao, L., McCallum, A.: Modeling relations and their mentions without labeled text. In: Balcázar, J.L., Bonchi, F., Gionis, A., Sebag, M. (eds.) ECML PKDD 2010. LNCS, vol. 6323, pp. 148–163. Springer, Heidelberg (2010). doi:10.1007/978-3-642-15939-8_10
10. Surdeanu, M., Tibshirani, J., Nallapati, R., Manning, C.D.: Multi-instance multi-label learning for relation extraction. In: The 2012 Joint Conference on Empirical Methods in Natural Language Processing and Computational Natural Language Learning, pp. 455–465. Association for Computational Linguistics, Stroudsburg (2012)
11. Xu, W., Hoffmann, R., Zhao, L., Grishman, R.: Filling knowledge base gaps for distant supervision of relation extraction. In: The 51st Annual Meeting of the Association for Computational Linguistics, pp. 665–670. Association for Computational Linguistics, Stroudsburg (2013)
12. Chen, Y., Geng, G.H., Jia, H.: Density center graph based weakly supervised classification algorithm. J. Comput. Eng. Appl. 6(51), 6–10 (2015)
13. Collobert, R., Weston, J., Bottou, L.: Natural language processing (almost) from scratch. J. Mach. Learn. Res. 12, 2493–2537 (2011)
14. Yih, W., He, X., Meek, C.: Semantic parsing for single- relation question answering. In: The Annual Meeting of the Association for Computational Linguistics, pp. 643–648 (2014)
15. Kim, Y.: Convolutional neural networks for sentence classification. arXiv preprint arXiv: 1408-5882 (2014)
16. Zou, Y.W., Gu, J.G., Fu, H.D.: EARES: medical entity and attribute extraction system based on relation annotation. Wuhan Univ. J. Nat. Sci. 21(2), 145–150 (2016)

Strategies and Challenges of Multilingual Information Retrieval on Health Forum

Ye Liang[(⊠)], Ying Qin, and Bing Fu

Department of Computer Science, Beijing Foreign Studies University,
Beijing 100089, China
{liangye,qinying,fub}@bfsu.edu.cn

Abstract. Multilingual information retrieval is very important to the persons who need to consolidate information from different languages posts and forums. However, it is not an easy job to find appropriate citations for a given context, especially for citations in different languages. In this paper, we define a novel computing framework of massive posts data and user behavior data to realize multilingual information retrieval and key technologies of multilingual information retrieval. This task is very challenging because the posts data are written in different languages and there exists a language gap when matching them. To tackle this problem, we propose the multilingual posts matching technology, source information handling technology, and personalized feed or smart feed technology. We evaluate the proposed methods based on a real dataset that contains Chinese posts data and English posts data. The results demonstrate that our proposed algorithms can outperform the conventional information retrieval scheme.

Keywords: Multilingual · Information retrieval · Health forum · Big data

1 Introduction

With the development of information technology, the user's requirement in information retrieval becomes greater diversification, so information searching and accessing is no longer limited to professional persons or professional books. At the same time, the users of a health forum are not only the information requester, but also the creator and disseminators of information. Internet users are more willing to send comments or forward other people's opinions on these forums [1]. They do consultation and know more in the interaction with friends. Their comments and forward constitute the entire operating environment of the forum. So that everyone is a publisher of the information and each message has the potential of thousands of readers [2].

Furthermore, Internet users may be not gotten enough information through their native language when they are collecting information from health forums. Therefore, they have to try to obtain more information from forum post written by non-native language [3, 4]. But as you known, it's very difficult and time consuming to read a great quantity of post written by non-native language which they haven't grasp skillfully to

© Springer International Publishing AG 2017
C. Xing et al. (Eds.): ICSH 2016, LNCS 10219, pp. 57–62, 2017.
DOI: 10.1007/978-3-319-59858-1_6

try to retrieve the key information from them. So, this is the biggest challenge to retrieve multilingual information on health forums [5, 6].

2 Analysis of the Key Technology

Based on the study of linguistics, information science, and library and information science, the key technology of multilingual information retrieval in this paper focuses on the real-time messages posted on the authority health forums in the world's major countries. By analyzing the massive posts and blogs of different information sources and language origins, we come up with a basic theory model and its algorithm on posts, which is capable of intelligent collection, quick access, deduplication, correction and integration with posts' backgrounds. Furthermore, we can find out connections between posts or blogs and posters' interest. So we can achieve a real-time and on-demand posts feed.

Therefore, the key problem in this paper is how to establish a mapping between real-time multi-source posts and potential readers in the times of big data. Based on the above analysis, the study of the key technology of multilingual information retrieval focuses on the multilingual problem, source information handling and decision-making of information feed.

2.1 Multilingual Problem

Wide coverage, high quality and authoritative and reliable contents are three basic attributes of high quality posts service. The project first makes a list of authority forums sites. The list contains various authority posts sources of the world's major languages, so we can get the real-time posts. Then based on the improved crawler technology combining with multilingual posts collection based on dictionary and corpora, we realize the multilingual posts recognition, editing and correlation matching technologies.

The multilingual information matching technology focuses on relationship of concept in various languages. Based on the pattern of the dictionary, the statistical sorting method is adopted to category the keywords. Or based on the pattern of the bilingual corpora, the mapping between bilingual corpora.

The difficulty of multilingual posts matching technology lies in the study of context disambiguation. And semantic correlations between keywords help to control the keyword disambiguation and reduce the semantic dimension.

2.2 Source Information Handling

The multilingual information collection problem is followed by the problem of source information handling. The key technologies in source information handling research contain network hot topic detection and tracking, topic recognition, topic classification, new event detection, posts report segmentation, identification of posts coverage correlation, topic tracking, automatic summarization generation, subject extraction and so on.

The improved simHash algorithm is adopted in our project to classify the posts topics. Not only deduplication of webs but the deletion of posts of low quality is realized. And the improved Naive Bayes Classifier is adopted in the information coverage segmentation.

As for topic classification, there are clear and consistent timing relations between the original event about the topic and its consecutive events. So it's an important evaluation metric of correlation judgment. Generally, the closer the time distance between posts coverage and events is, the more probability of them belonging to the same topic. The difficulty is to distinguish between different events of the same topic. As the same topic triggered by different events often reappears, what the topic describes is the generality shared by all the similar events. The biggest difference between different events is that occurred time and place is not consistent, the characters and organization can be quite different. A feature set mainly containing this type of nouns is meaningful for identifying different events.

2.3 Effective Decision-Making of Information Feed

The word 'feed' means that the reader get the posts without direct involvement. For different users, the posts fed in the traditional way is classified by user types. So users of the same category get the same posts. That is, the posts fed is not sorted and selected according to users' interests. And time factor seems to have no influence on the result of posts feed. The posts can't reflect the popular information and latest hot topics about which people are concerned most.

So personalized feed or smart feed is a key problem this paper tries to solve. It can increase users' satisfaction with posts feed if we can develop different feed strategies when confronting with different users. The aim of personalized service is to feed posts of high quality in order to improve user experience and the application's competitiveness and its appeal. Thus, personalized feed needs to record and analyze user behaviors to understand and predict users' interests. And then it can provide customized services.

There are two kinds of users' interests: long-term and short-term. We need to build s corresponding user model according to historical information about user access and historical user behaviors. The system will feed the posts to users according to the user model when it detects a new event. And then it records the user's browsing and stores it in history information. So we can update user model later. Also, the analysis of user behaviors can be applied to the posts feed where users have similar request.

In the implementation, the method of user feedback is adopted as means of accuracy improvement of posts feed. That is, the users' first selections of posts are inputs of the second posts feed. It can be seen as a user interaction, which may control the ambiguity of multilingual information retrieval. At the same time, the residence time of the user on a page and the content size are regarded as an input of user interaction. So we can calculate the conformity of the content, which is the input of next selection of posts feed. Tracking user feedback in the above iterative way provides the personalized service with theoretical basis.

3   Framework of Multilingual Information Retrieval

We need to break through in the fields of key technologies framework of multilingual information retrieval, computing framework of massive posts data and user behavior data to realize multilingual information retrieval and key technologies of multilingual information retrieval.

The posts items and trajectory information of user behavior involved in the process of multilingual information retrieval belong to the field of massive information. Take trajectory information of user behavior as an example, suppose that each user reads average 30 posts items a day, it will create thirty items of trajectory information. That is, it will create more than 10000 items of trajectory information. Similarly, one million users will create 10 billion items of trajectory information. It's impossible to analyze user behavior from so large amount of data.

Thus, the computing framework is adopted to cope with the connection between tables with massive data. The preliminary research framework is shown in Fig. 1.

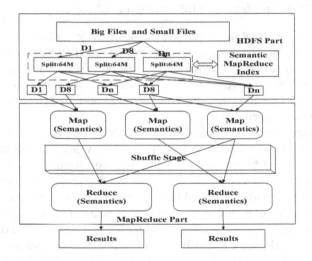

Fig. 1. Blood estimation work flow

The project tries to analyze the most effective network computing framework based on the existing Internet popular framework of Google MapReduce, Hadoop MapReduce, Twister, Hadoop, Hadoop++, Hadoop DB of Yale University and Spark of University of California at Berkeley. By analyzing the internal structure of Hadoop++, the method of semantic computing is adopted to improve the query accuracy and its efficiency under the MapReduce framework. By analyzing the principle of Twister and Hadoop framework, the new framework of massive data computing is adopted to cope with the problem of iterative and loop calculation. By reprocessing the file partitioning mechanism, the capacity of Split is decreased from 64M to 1M to improve the ability of massive small file processing. The phase of Shuffle has the most effect on the computing efficiency in the whole network computing system. It's a bottleneck of the computing. And to deal with the bottleneck, both the semantics scheduling technique and semantics fault-tolerant technique are adopted to realize the effective task scheduling. So we can improve the ability of response and fault-tolerant disposal.

4   Experimental Result

4.1   Experimental Preparation

Compare the efficiency of conventional information retrieval computation and multilingual information retrieval simulation calculation based on big data with Hadoop MapReduce. The content is several multilingual posts wrote in English and Chinese.

In the simulation experiment, 8 virtual machines are simulated through cloud platforms CloudSim. One of the virtual machines serves as Name node, and other three virtual machines serve as Data node. Chinese or English post data sets, with 100M, 200M, 300M, 400M, 500M posts respectively, are used as the testing dataset.

4.2   Analysis of Simulation Results

Figure 2 shows the simulation results in conventional information retrieval scheme and multilingual information retrieval scheme.

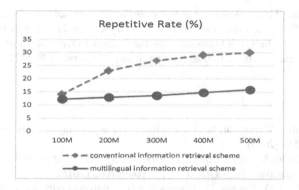

Fig. 2. The simulation experiment results

From Fig. 2, as the dataset's scale increases gradually, repetitive rate in feeding posts is increasing, and it shows an accelerating trend. The main reason is that if there is more posts, there will be more difficult to recognize the difference among posts. In addition, as can be seen from the diagram, using multilingual information retrieval scheme, repetitive rate is lower than using the conventional information retrieval scheme, which explains that multilingual information matching technology could give more help to distinguish the similar posts in different languages.

5 Conclusion

Reading posts is one of the basic demands of forum users. And mobile phone reading is the most popular way of reading among youngsters. If the traditional information retrieval of no difference is transformed into the personalized one, it will be widespread in the youngsters. Besides, due to the information retrieval and selection as a premise and a network flooded with massive information, it's a time consuming and labor intensive process to select post manually. Also, information like the forum posts require high real-time. Manual-selection-based information retrieval decreases the availability of the posts. The cycle of selection, translation and retrieval will be longer especially when the posts is in foreign languages. It also decreases the value of the posts. Therefore, the multilingual contents are rarely involved in the current retrieval.

The multilingual information retrieval provides people capable of multilingual reading with multilingual, smart and customized services. It reduces the information retrieval time. And it's a source supplement of information retrieval in forums, due to its vast posts sources, massive information and reliability and timeliness. Also, it is valuable in helping promote the current forum using its technologies. Besides, the relevant result of our study can be applied to network information retrievals, which will be a theoretical basis of applications like network anti-terrorism, public opinion research and research progress tracking.

Acknowledgments. This work was supported in part by the National Social Science Foundation of China (No. 15CTQ028, No. 14@ZH036), Social Science Foundation of Beijing (No. 15SHA002), Scientific Research Foundation for the Returned Overseas Chinese Scholars, and Young Faculty Research Fund of Beijing Foreign Studies University (2015JT008).

References

1. Burton, R., Collins-Thompson, K.: User behavior in asynchronous slow search. In: SIGIR 2016, pp. 345–354 (2016)
2. Mehrotra, R., Bhattacharya, P., Yilmaz, E.: Uncovering task based behavioral heterogeneities in online search behavior. In: SIGIR 2016, pp. 1049–1052 (2016)
3. Raviv, H., Kurland, O., Carmel, D.: Document retrieval using entity-based language models. In: SIGIR 2016, pp. 65–74 (2016)
4. Kumar, B.A.: Profound survey on cross language information retrieval methods (CLIR). In: Conference on Advanced Computing & Communication Technologies, pp. 64–68 (2012)
5. Tomassetti, F., Rizzo, G., Troncy, R.: Cross language spotter: a library for detecting relations in polyglot frameworks. In: WWW 2014, pp. 583–586 (2014)
6. Yuan,D., Mitra, P.: Cross language indexing and retrieval of the cypriot digital antiquities repository. In: DocEng2013, pp. 235–236 (2013)

Health Data Analysis and Management, Healthcare Intelligent Systems and Clinical Practice

Part II Data Analysis and Management, Healthcare Intelligent Systems and Clinical Practice

SilverLink: Developing an International Smart and Connected Home Monitoring System for Senior Care

Lubaina Maimoon[1]([✉]), Joshua Chuang[1], Hongyi Zhu[2], Shuo Yu[2], Kuo-Shiuan Peng[2], Rahul Prayakarao[1], Jie Bai[3], Daniel Zeng[3], Shu-Hsing Li[4], Hsinmin Lu[4], and Hsinchun Chen[2]

[1] Caduceus Intelligence Corporation, Tucson, AZ, USA
lubainamaimoon@gmail.com, joshua.chuang@gmail.com,
rahulprayakarao@gmail.com
[2] Artificial Intelligence Lab, University of Arizona, Tucson, AZ, USA
{zhuhy,shuoyu,kspeng}@email.arizona.edu, hchen@eller.arizona.edu
[3] Chinese Academy of Science, Beijing, China
baijie2013@ia.ac.cn, zengdaniel@outlook.com
[4] National Taiwan University, Taipei, Taiwan
taiwanshli@management.ntu.edu.tw, luim@ntu.edu.tw

Abstract. Due to increased longevity, there has been a significant growth in the aging population world over. Caring for this burgeoning class has become a pressing challenge faced by many developed and emerging countries, including the US (the aging baby boomer) and China (the reverse 4-2-1 family pyramid due to one child policy). Despite failing health, most senior citizens prefer to live independently at home and hence the focus of current healthcare technologies has shifted from traditional clinical care to "at-home" care for the senior citizens. We propose to develop SilverLink, a system that is unique in its smart and connected technologies and will offer: (1) affordable and non-invasive home-based mobile health technologies for monitoring health-related motion and daily activities; (2) advanced mobile health analytics algorithms for fall detection, health status progression monitoring, and health anomaly detection and alert; and (3) a comprehensive health activity portal for reporting user activity and health status and for engaging family members. This review discusses the SilverLink system in detail along with some of the technical challenges faced during the development of this system and future opportunities.

Keywords: Health big data · Home health monitoring · Health progression monitoring · Senior care · Gait analysis

1 Introduction

Aging is the reality of the future world. With improvements in healthcare, life expectancy has drastically improved in the last decade. Demographic trends indicate that the aging population world over is growing at an enormous rate with more than 20% of the population in the US expected to be above the age of 65 in 2060 [1]. This is important because aging has profound consequences on a broad range of economic, political and

C. Xing et al. (Eds.): ICSH 2016, LNCS 10219, pp. 65–77, 2017.
DOI: 10.1007/978-3-319-59858-1_7

social processes. As more and more people enter old age, it has become a priority to promote their wellbeing as aging is often accompanied by several chronic conditions and susceptibility to injuries due to cognitive impairment and loss of motor control. According to the U.S. Centers for Disease Control and Prevention, one out of every three adults (above the age of 65) falls each year and these falls are among the leading cause of fatal and non-fatal injuries. In 2013 alone, the number of emergency cases (due to falls) equaled 2.5 million with more than 700,000 hospitalized 25,000 dead [2]. In 2013, the direct medical costs of falls were $34 billion and these costs will only accelerate as more and more senior citizens opt to "age at home" with no functional support system in place to aid it. Moreover, the responsibility will now lie on family members and caregivers as the number of dependent individuals increase but the number of people who can support them will either remain the same or decrease due to self or government imposed family planning measures. In China, the previously 1-child and now 2-child policy has resulted in a significant increase in the dependent to caregiver ratio. Family caregiving is both emotionally and physically demanding and is generally unpaid. According to a study, the estimated value of this unpaid care is about $257M dollars annually [3]. As most senior citizens prefer to "age in place," the number of older adults living alone continues to increase with at least one out of three non-institutionalized senior citizens living alone [4]. Independent living (e.g., private households) will be an important housing option for the future, particularly for the newly aged [5] and the applications of in-home monitoring technologies will have enormous potential for assuaging the emotional and monetary burden on caregivers/family members.

To provide older adults with the required level of independence in terms of care, methods to detect cognitive and physical decline that put them at risk must be in place. There are several potential technologies under development for remote health monitoring. These technologies range from in-house lifestyle monitoring to fall detection and monitoring of health vitals such as blood pressure, etc. [6]. The major limitations of current products are the high cost of technology, lack of flexibility in use, and limited one-dimensional data collection and analytics to "intelligently" monitor health status of senior citizens at-home. Even with the recent developments, there is a need for an affordable but smart and non-invasive health monitoring system. The proposed system, SilverLink (SL), aims at developing, evaluating, and commercializing an easy to use, all encompassing smart and connected home monitoring system that will allow users to have extended functionalities at a more affordable cost.

2 Literature Review and Related Systems

2.1 Remote Health Monitoring Techniques

Remote health monitoring has broadly widened its scope in the last few years. Remote monitoring (via telemedicine), previously employed as means for a follow up patient consult is now a means to support prevention (of falls, etc.), medication adherence, early diagnosis, disease management and home rehabilitation. Using remote health monitoring, especially for those suffering from chronic conditions and in need of long-term care, could lead to a significant reduction in healthcare costs by avoiding unnecessary hospitalizations and ensuring that those in need of urgent care receive it sooner. Latest developments in micro- and nanotechnologies as well as in information processing and wireless communication offer, today, the possibility for smart miniaturization and non-invasive biomedical measurement as well as for wearable sensing, processing and communication. Remote health monitoring systems are designed to gather data about patients' status and relay it efficiently to healthcare providers/caregivers/physicians on a regular basis. They pave a path for communicating with patients (or users) beyond the acute care setting. Most such devices/systems fall under one or more of the following sub categories: mobility tracking, patient support portals, and advanced health analytics.

2.1.1 Mobility Tracking

Mobility tracking in terms of health monitoring is capturing human motion or move-ments. The manner in which a person performs a physical activity is highly indicative of her/his health and quality of life. Quantification and reliable measurement of daily physical activity can allow an effective assessment of a person's daily activities as well as the effects of numerous medical conditions and treatments, especially in people suffering from chronic diseases such as arthritis, cardiovascular or neurodegenerative diseases that can often affect gait and mobility [7]. Many researchers have focused their attention towards gait analysis for health progression monitoring and fall detection. However, due to technological constraints such as the need to use multiple wearable sensors for accurate data gathering in case of gait analysis have resulted in limiting this critical research to the laboratory with no real-life applications in place.

2.1.2 Health Activity Portals and Support

Health and mobility restrictions often result in shrinking a senior citizen's physical and social reach. Digital technology has an obvious role to play here by connecting people virtually when being together is difficult or impossible. Research shows that "persuasive technology" [8] in the form of personal messages, frequent communication via photos, videos, and other means can often help motivate people to change their attitudes, and in turn better manage their health. For example, portals such as DiabeticLink provide a platform for diabetics to track and easily visualize health data on the portal and improve health outcomes by monitoring how one health factor can affect another [9].

2.1.3 Advanced Health Analytics

With the advancements in sensor technology, it is now possible to collect data about any person in a home-based environment. Data (for healthcare) collected can range from movement of objects (e.g., displacement of a pillbox) to human motion (e.g., walking, jogging, sitting). In-depth analysis of the collected data patterns can prove useful in predicting patient behavior and health outcomes, enabling the development of a more personalized healthcare solution [10]. One limitation of existing tools is that they lack monitoring capabilities for progression of frailty (slow and natural health deterioration) in older adults. The existing solutions to home health monitoring are divided into two main categories:

(1) *Personalized Emergency Response Systems (PERS):* One of the most widely used technology-based home care solutions today, PERS provides an easy way to summon assistance in case of an emergency. Advanced PERS also possess fall detection and fall prediction capabilities; however, they do not provide all the components of home health monitoring, e.g., activity monitoring, medicine reminders, etc. Examples of these devices include Alert 1 and Philips Medical Alert System. In addition, Internet-connected fitness wristbands (e.g., FitBit) and health-monitoring smart watches (e.g., Apple Watch) are gaining traction with the youth. Despite their emerging popularity, such devices do not target home care or activity monitoring for the aging population.

(2) *Home-Use Monitoring with Sensors:* Some of the more mature but basic home monitoring systems such as home security systems (*e.g.*, ADT home security) and home video surveillance (e.g., Nest Cam) do not adopt or leverage advanced multi-sensor technologies or cloud-based intelligent analytics services. Some Smart Home researchers used object sensors with pressure sensors on the floor to recognize users' daily activities, which is not easily applicable in real home settings [11].

Thus, we propose a system called SilverLink that is unique in its capabilities and encompasses all the aspects of remote monitoring, i.e., mobility tracking, lifestyle monitoring, online health support and advanced analytics. SilverLink aims to overcome both, technological and functional challenges faced by existing remote monitoring tools.

3   System Design

3.1   SilverLink Architecture

The SilverLink system developed with funding support from National Science Foundation (NSF), US, consists of both hardware and software components. The hardware components include multiple motion sensors, a gateway and a wearable sensor with an SOS alarm button. The software components consist of data collection API, a database, an analytics engine and a web portal. The overall service architecture is shown in Fig. 1. The SL system consists of 4 object sensors and 1 human (wearable) sensor. The object sensors can be attached to relevant household objects to indicate user activity or health status, e.g., pillbox (indicating medication compliance), refrigerator door (indicating food intake), etc. The wearable human sensor can be used to capture different human motions, such as walking, falling, etc. A pre-configured gateway is designed to use BLE and 3G/WiFi communication techniques to receive and transmit data collected from the sensors to the Datacenter and into our analytics engine.

Our advanced analytics engine processes the data to make deductions based on pattern recognition and in turn generate notifications/alerts when a shift in pattern is detected. The wearable device with the SOS button can be activated (by the user) to alert a response team in case of an emergency. The SilverLink web portal will also provide a platform (on devices such as laptops, tablets, mobile phones, etc.) to visualize the health information collected by the sensors.

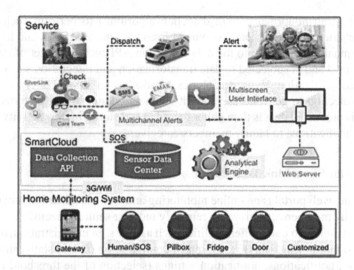

Fig. 1. SilverLink Architecture: Hardware (Sensors/Gateway), Software (Analytics/Portal), and Services

3.2 Hardware Design for Home Activity Sensors and Gateway

SilverLink uses two types of activity sensors: (1) object sensors and (2) human sensors. Both types of sensors have high sensitivity, high frequency of data sampling and are comprised of accelerometers and gyroscopes. Each sensor communicates wirelessly via Bluetooth. It periodically emits signals to indicate sensor status and to synchronize with other components of the monitoring system. Because of Bluetooth, the range on the sensors is about 10–12 m. The sensor, powered by a coin cell battery, is enclosed in a light but durable casing with an attachment mechanism so it can be fixed onto a variety of different objects. For human motion monitoring, the sensor can be easily attached to a user's belt/keychain or worn as a pendant. The home gateway is an Android Smartphone with Bluetooth, 3G and WiFi capabilities.

3.3 Data Collection API and Activity Database

The data collection API is used to accept data from the different sensors placed in a user's home. The datacenter is configured to store raw data collected from activity sensors and sent via the gateway. Examples of the types of data stored in the tables include gateway, sensor and system information; raw sensor log data; processed data representing user activities; and web portal management data such as user login and profile, links, notifications, etc.

3.4 Process Design for Advanced Analytics Engine

SilverLink's novel analytics engine is configured to process and analyze data obtained by other components of the system. Accordingly, the analytics engine employs an algorithm (e.g., an abnormal pattern detection algorithm) to perform such tasks as advanced pattern recognition. Data is sourced from the remote sensors and transmitted through the monitoring system to the data collection API such that a set of raw sensor data is generated and is subjected to data transformation and integration steps for noise reduction and sanitization. Various analytics approaches including pattern recognition and signal detection to generate user activity data and define signal patterns are then used and this processed data is then either recorded and stored in user activity tables or will trigger notifications to family members/caregivers.

3.5 Design for SilverLink Web Portal

The SilverLink web portal is an online monitoring and data visualization tool designed to allow family members/caregivers to remotely monitor senior citizens.

The SilverLink web portal offers utilities such as user sign in/registration, user dashboard to view monitoring data (Fig. 2), sensor configuration (sensor status and location of the sensor), notifications, notification settings (selection of the threshold for notification/alert generation) and administrative options (adding or editing a new user profile). The web portal provides password-protected access to registered users and is accessible from computers, tablets or smartphones. The portal also generates alerts, (via text/email) in case of activity pattern anomalies and; a summary page, which displays the daily average activity count over a period of 7 days. This summary is sent out weekly via email to keep the user/caregivers updated. The organizational dashboard can effectively reduce operational cost by allocating more attention to high-risk elderlies.

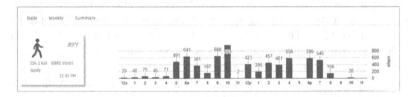

Fig. 2. SilverLink's user dashboard displaying a user's activity summary for the day

Once our hardware and software development was complete, the next step was a to perform a comprehensive system evaluation in order to determine how the system fares in real world settings. Our evaluation included extensive internal and external testing procedures, which are discussed in detail in the following sections.

4　Preliminary System Evaluation

In order to determine the technical feasibility of our system, we designed and conducted a user study, which was approved by University of Arizona's Institutional Review Board. The main objective of the study, its methodology and results are as follows:

4.1   Objective

The aim of this study was to evaluate the SilverLink system based on several parameters including form factor, user comfort, technical feasibility and system stability to uncover potential opportunities for system improvement and gather data for advancing our analytics research.

4.2   System Evaluation Methodology

This study was conducted in two phases. For the first phase of system evaluation (or internal testing), we used the following usability testing methodologies: expert review and remote testing to evaluate factors such as the operating distance between the Gateway and the sensors (range), battery life, data transmission rate, data loss rate, system errors, stability of the portal, the capabilities of the analytics engine and other system heuristics. This internal testing was carried out in the US, Taiwan and China to determine system compatibility with different networks in varied settings.

For the second phase or external testing, we screened and selected candidates that best matched our target population. The participants were asked to participate in a short pre-test interview (qualitative) before we installed the SilverLink system in their houses and then a longer post-test interview (qualitative) after 4–6 weeks of continuously using the system. Both, the pre and post-test questionnaires were designed to gauge user's interest and comfort in using the SilverLink system.

5   Preliminary Findings

5.1   Internal Testing

As mentioned previously, the internal testing was carried out by our teams in the US, Taiwan and China. Each team tested 10–15 sets in different settings with randomly selected participants. Participants included domain experts, students, working professionals and retired citizens. Each randomly selected user was asked to install and use the SilverLink system (following set guidelines) for at least a month and provide feedback on different aspects of the system as discussed under system evaluation methodology. Some of the technical issues reported and resolved during this evaluation phase are summarized below.

5.1.1   Improvements in Sensor Functionality

During our research into the home health monitoring market, we realized that battery life is a major cause for concern among most devices serving this segment. Even a simple step counter like Fitbit has to be charged once every week. During our internal testing, we faced similar battery issues with our sensors. To ensure the sustainable use of our system in the field, we strived to extend the battery life of the sensors.

Most human sensors on the market either only store and transmit the summarized data (e.g., step numbers and total distances), which doesn't support detailed analytics;

or continuously stream movement data to the cloud for analytics which drains battery quickly. We aimed to balance data granularity and power consumption in our use cases. To begin with, we examined the rate of power consumption at different stages of sensor functionality, such as configuration, transmission, etc. We then analyzed and designed optimal battery consumption procedures at each stage and identified several reasons for a high initial battery consumption (2–3/10 days for human/object sensors). These were continuous BLE (Bluetooth Low Energy) connection (also known as streaming mode), incompatible firmware update and download of unnecessary stationary data. To address these issues, we implemented, in our sensors, a 'logging mode' that only triggers data transmission from the sensor to the gateway when a connection is established between the two. In addition, by applying the 'any motion detection' logic, the battery life of human sensor increased to 4–5 weeks and that of the object sensors increased to 10 weeks. Lastly, we increased the BLE advertising interval to further extend object sensor's battery life to more than 4 months. Among other improvements, to optimize sensor sensitivity, we implemented a filter to reduce noise from picking up undesirable events. The next section discusses the development of the gateway app.

5.1.2   Improvements in Gateway App

For our gateway, we selected a low-cost Android smartphone with 3G, WiFi and BLE capabilities that allows development of a customized SilverLink app with sensor's Android SDK (Software Development Kit). SL's gateway app is run as a foreground service to boost its robustness as select background services are terminated by the Android system when low on resources. One drawback of the device is the low number (2–4) of concurrent BLE connections that can be established at any point of time. To work around this constraint, we employed a rotating connection mechanism to ensure that all 5 sensors could connect to the gateway.

We also found that our app would not attempt to reconnect to a WiFi network automatically upon a disconnection. To resolve this, we developed a mechanism to automatically re-establish WiFi connectivity if it was dropped. Wi-Fi availability and stability is one challenge we faced especially in Taiwan and China. Our Android phone-based gateway can utilize 3G to solve this connectivity issue and hence we are exploring local 3G options for our next version.

In a real world setting, our system should require very little user involvement. For this purpose, our gateway has been designed with a built-in auto-update. The gateway also has an auto crash report system and can reset itself, should any error occur.

5.1.3   Improvements in Battery Gauge/Meter

Another major concern with IoT devices is inaccurate indication of the battery percentage (charge remaining). This issue occurs because the battery percentage meter for an IoT device is voltage-based. The IoT system converts the effective working voltage to a percentage. However, the working voltage is sensitive to the ambient temperature. Thus, the battery percentage is unstable and non-linear. To solve this, we measured the voltage of a battery under different temperature conditions for the same period of time and used linear regression to generate a mapping table, which is used to map the voltage percentage to a stable and linear value in different temperatures.

After completing extensive internal testing, we moved to the second phase of our system evaluation. The results of this study are summarized in the section below.

5.2   SilverLink US Evaluation

The external usability study was conducted with 6 participants that matched our study criteria. These participants were in the age group of 76–89 years and were living in independent housing, either alone or with their spouse. Our selected participants suffered from various health conditions ranging from arthritis, fibromyalgia, sepsis due to a prior infection, Parkinson's disease and other heart conditions. This made them a suitable fit for our usability study.

5.2.1   User Feedback
Before setting up the system for our participant (user), we conducted a pretest interview which gave us information about their daily routines, use of alternate home monitoring systems and general level of comfort with smartphones, iPads and tablets. We also asked them about their biggest fear when it came to living alone. This helped us assess the need for a system like SilverLink and its best possible use for each individual participant.

At the end of 6 weeks, we conducted another round of interviews to find out what the users thought about the SilverLink system. The questions addressed several aspects of the system including system design, user comfort, portal usability, etc. The initial feedback that we received was as follows:

- 6/6 users said the sensors are light weight, non-obtrusive and comfortable to wear 24*7
- 6/6 users said the human sensor is better designed than their PERs system
- 6/6 users said that an SOS button is a must-have for them
- 3/6 users said they would use the system for home security in addition to health monitoring
- 3/6 users suggested implementing GPS on the human sensor
- 2/6 users said that the system was useful in monitoring sleeping patterns
- 2/6 users said that activity monitoring (using object sensors) was not a must-have feature whereas gait monitoring using the human sensor was.
- 1/6 users said the device was useful for monitoring eating habits
- 1/6 users said that the SilverLink portal motivated her to set goals and be more active

During this study, no family members or caregivers were involved due to which it was not possible to accurately judge the usefulness of the entire system (including the online activity portal). We aim target participants including family members and retirement community staff members in the next phase of the study.

In terms of technical feasibility, the SilverLink system faced two major issues: (1) the loss of WiFi connectivity when using a public network and (2) unexpectedly low battery life (2–3 weeks) of the human sensor when used continuously.

5.3 SilverLink China Evaluation

To evaluate the effectiveness and robustness of the system outside the US, we conducted a user study in China as well. The 7 participants (users) were mostly IT technicians who have senior family members living with them but have never used home health monitoring devices before. We selected families with several different house floor plans and home settings, to ensure that different conditions have been considered in the test.

5.3.1 User Feedback

Overall, the users were satisfied with the system. The feedback received was:

- 5/7 users said that the system "lets them know about their family members whenever they want"
- 4/7 users said that is was "fit for seniors who live alone"
- 3/7 users said the dashboard charts were difficult to understand
- 2/7 users said that sensor range was a problem in houses bigger than 100 m^2

Other suggestions made included extending the system functionality to record outdoor activities, changing the human sensor from a pendant into a wristband (5/7) and extending the remote functionality to cater to both senior and child care (1/7).

Our immediate next steps, based on the results of the user study, are to improve sensor battery life and incorporate the SOS (PERs) functionality. We will also continue testing our system with a larger group of people including family members/caregivers of senior citizens and further our mobile sensor research on fall detection and activity of daily living recognition. The preliminary results of this research are described in Sect. 6.

6   Preliminary Mobile Sensor Research and Results

6.1 Fall Detection Research Design and Preliminary Findings

We conducted a preliminary study on designing a fall detection system using the SiverLink human sensor. This sensor contains a tri-axial accelerometer to track the user's movements and send acceleration signals to the gateway. Analytic algorithms were used to aggregate the signals to high-level parameters (e.g., walking speed and step count) and make meaningful inferences.

A fall is an event, which results in a person coming to rest inadvertently on the ground or floor or other lower level [1]. Three phases can be identified during a fall event: collapse, impact, and inactivity [12]. There have been studies on fall detection attempting to capture the features for one or more of the three phases, by measuring maximum acceleration, vertical velocity, posture change, etc. [13, 14]. However, most of the prior studies used threshold-based or classifier-based systems based on signal processing or fall specific features, which did not take the time precedence of the three phases into account. The absence or order change of any phases may lead to different scenarios other than fall events. For instance, missing the inactivity phase may indicate that the fall is of no or minimal damage. Furthermore, prior studies fixed the sensor orientation and position on human body for their experiments, which is a void assumption in real world scenarios. Real users typically wear the human sensor in any arbitrary orientation. To resolve the two issues, we proposed a fall detection system based on hidden Markov models (HMMs) with sensor orientation calibration techniques. HMMs are a temporal pattern recognition models that characterizes human motor states (e.g., standing upright still, falling, impact, lying down still, etc.). Figure 3 illustrates the human motor states during a simulated fall event.

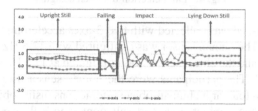

Fig. 3. Human motor states during a simulated fall event

Each HMM can characterize a single category of fall events or normal activities, e.g., fall forward, or walking. We construct multiple HMMs to model various categories of those activities, including fall forward, fall backward, fall laterally left, fall laterally right, quiet standing, quiet sitting, quiet lying, walking, stand-up, sit-down, lie-down, and get-up from bed. To evaluate our system, we collected signal samples from five student volunteers (average age: 27 years). Five sensors were attached to each volunteer at five positions on human body, including neck, chest, waist, left side and right side. Each sensor was considered a separate event (we did not use multiple sensors for one event at a time). We collected 100 simulated fall events and 185 normal activities. We evaluated our model in ten-fold cross validation and achieved a sensitivity of 0.990 and a specificity of 0.984, which means only one missed fall for every 100 falls, and less than two false alarms for every 100 normal activities. Our next step is to evaluate our system using real fall events, and deploy our system to real users, to further validate its performance and effectiveness.

6.2   Activity of Daily Living (ADL) Recognition Research Design and Findings

Some researchers introduced Activity of Daily Living, such as functional mobility, and food preparing, to evaluate senior's self-care ability. Our preliminary research is focused on evaluating how the use of object sensors with a human sensor (with an advanced algorithm) can give us a better understanding of a user's ADL and help in ADL recognition. We proposed a deep learning based approach (see Fig. 4) to process raw accelerometer readings with SilverLink's human and object sensors and extract the ADLs. The approach utilized CNN layers to extract locally dependent sensor interactions and a sequence-to-sequence Recurrent Neural Networks (RNN) layer to extract ADLs from the recognized interaction sequences.

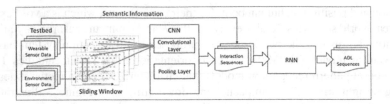

Fig. 4. Fall detection research design

The research test-bed was collected with two 3-axes accelerometers in a controlled home environment. The human sensor was configured with 12.5 Hz sampling rate and a sensitivity of ±4G and the object sensor was configured at 12.5 Hz sampling rate with a sensitivity of ±2G. The participants wore the human sensor as a pendant. In these settings, we collected four target human-object interactions (using object sensors placed on refrigerator/restroom/cabinet door and salt containers/pillboxes), including pull, push, pick up, and put down. In total, the data set is separated into the training set with 3600 data frames, the validation set with 600 data frames, and the Test set with 600 data frames. 1000 ADL sequences were bootstrapped from these data. According to the location information of the object sensors, each interaction in these sequences was labeled with the following four ADLs: medication, food intake, personal hygiene, and no activity. The training set, validation set, and test set has 800, 100, and 100 sequences.

6.2.1 Preliminary Findings

For interaction extraction task, we evaluate our CNN against SVM and kNN. The accuracy of CNN method was 99.5%, which exceeded the accuracy level of the baseline method SVM with RBF (98.36%) and kNN (k = 1) (96.42%). We compared the label-wise accuracy for the ADL recognition task against a 4-hidden-state HMM model with 2000 EM iterations. The result showed that with only 4 hidden nodes and 100 training epochs, RNN reached the similar accuracy level (46.57%) as HMM (48.71%). When we increased the number of RNN hidden nodes to 128, the accuracy increased to 61.81%. Overall, our deep learning (CNN + RNN) approach is a viable framework to recognize ADLs from raw sensor readings without manual feature identification and extraction.

7   Conclusion

There is a growing need for a smart and connected home health monitoring system that reduces manual effort and makes aging at home easier and safer for senior citizens. Our current research has helped validate the need for such a system and provided improvement opportunities both in terms of social and technical feasibility. The next step will be to conduct further user experience research in the US, China and Taiwan (with over 150 participants in total) in order to obtain further customer validation and determine system enhancement opportunities. We will also continue to improve hardware and software functionalities such as battery life, SOS alarm design, system stability, and data visualization on the SilverLink web portal.

Acknowledgements. This work is supported in part by the University of Arizona Artificial Intelligence Lab and Caduceus Intelligence Corporation, funded by the National Science Foundation (IIP-1622788) and the National Taiwan University (NTUH). We wish to acknowledge our collaborators in the U.S., Taiwan and China for their research support.

Dr. Hsinchun Chen declares a financial interest in Caduceus Intelligence Corporation, which owns the intellectual property involved in this research. This interest has been properly disclosed to the University of Arizona Institutional Review Committee and is managed in accordance with its conflict of interest policies.

References

1. World Health Organization. Ageing, & Life Course Unit. WHO global report on falls prevention in older age. World Health Organization (2008)
2. CDC National Safety Council. Report on Injuries in America (2003). http://www.nsc.org/library/report_injury_usa.htm. Accessed 2004
3. Toseland, R.W., Smith, G., McCallion, P.: Family caregivers of the frail elderly. In: Gitterman, A. (ed.) Handbook of Social Work Practice with Vulnerable and Resilient Populations. Columbia University, New York (2001)
4. Cannuscio, C., Block, J., Kawachi, I.: Social capital and successful aging: the role of senior housing. Ann. Intern. Med. **139**(5 Pt 2), 395–399 (2003)
5. Mann, W.C., Marchant, T., Tomita, M., Fraas, L., Stanton, K., Care, M.J.: Elder acceptance of health monitoring devices in the home. Winter **3**(2), 91–98 (2002)
6. Brownsell, S.J., Bradley, D.A., Bragg, R., Catlin, P., Carlier, J.: Do community alarm users want telecare? J. Telemed. Telecare **6**(4), 199–204 (2000)
7. Najafi, B., Aminian K., Paraschiv-Ionescu, A., Loew, F., Büla C.J., Robert, P.: Ambulatory system for human motion analysis using a kinematic sensor: monitoring of daily physical activity in the elderly. IEEE Trans. Biomed. Eng. **50**(6) (2003)
8. Fogg, B.J.: Persuasive Technology: Using Computers to Change What We Think and Do. Morgan Kaufmann Publishers, San Francisco (2002)
9. Chuang, J., et al.: DiabeticLink: an Integrated and Intelligent cyber-enabled health social platform for diabetic patients. In: Zheng, X., Zeng, D., Chen, H., Zhang, Y., Xing, C., Neill, Daniel B. (eds.) ICSH 2014. LNCS, vol. 8549, pp. 63–74. Springer, Cham (2014). doi: 10.1007/978-3-319-08416-9_7
10. Cortada, J., Gordon, D., Lenihan, B.: Advanced analytics in healthcare. In: Strome/Healthcare Healthcare Analytics for Quality and Performance Improvement, pp. 183–203. Web (2013)
11. Krishnan, N.C., Cook, D.J.: Activity recognition on streaming sensor data. Pervasive Mobile Comput. **10**, 138–154 (2014)
12. Lan, M., Nahapetian, A., Vahdatpour, A., Au, L., Kaiser, W., Sarrafzadeh, M.: SmartFall: an automatic fall detection system based on subsequence matching for the SmartCane. In: Proceedings of the Fourth International Conference on Body Area Networks, p. 8 (2009)
13. Bourke, A.K., Klenk, J., Schwickert, L., Aminian, K., Ihlen, E.A., Mellone, S., Becker, C.: Fall detection algorithms for real-world falls harvested from lumbar sensors in the elderly population: a machine learning approach. In: 2016 IEEE 38th Annual International Conference of the Engineering in Medicine and Biology Society (EMBC), pp. 3712–3715 (2016)
14. Lee, J.K., Robinovitch, S.N., Park, E.J.: Inertial sensing-based pre-impact detection of falls involving near-fall scenarios. IEEE Trans. Neural Syst. Rehabil. Eng. **23**(2), 258–266 (2015)

HKDP: A Hybrid Knowledge Graph Based Pediatric Disease Prediction System

Penghe Liu[1(✉)], Xiaoqing Wang[3], Xiaoping Sun[2], Xi Shen[1],
Xu Chen[1], Yuzhong Sun[1(✉)], and Yanjun Pan[1]

[1] State Key Laboratory of Computer Architecture,
Institute of Computing Technology, Chinese Academy of Sciences,
Beijing, China
{liupenghe, yuzhongsun}@ict.ac.cn
[2] Key Lab of Intelligent Information Processing, Chinese Academy of Sciences,
Beijing, China
[3] Beijing Chao-Yang Hospital Affiliated to Capital Medical University,
Beijing, China

Abstract. In this paper, we present a clinically pediatric disease prediction system based on a new efficient hybrid knowledge graph. Firstly, we automatically extract a set of triples by modeling and analyzing 1454 clinically pediatric cases, building a weighted knowledge graph based Naïve Bayes. Secondly, to extract new prediction opportunities from heterogeneous data sources, we model and analyze both classically professional pediatrics textbooks and clinical experiences of pediatric doctors respectively in order to derive prediction rules. Thirdly, we mix up those rules with the weighted knowledge graph we built to propose a new hybrid knowledge graph which can carry on both the Bayesian reasoning and the logic calculation at the same time. Fourthly, in term of that hybrid knowledge graph, we further design a new multi-label classifier based on the well-known Bayesian Ranking for the disease prediction. Finally, we implement such a hybrid knowledge graph based disease pediatric prediction system (HKDP) which uses the descriptions of the patients' symptoms as the inputs so as to return the predicted candidates of diseases for a child. In our experiments, the comparisons with classical prediction methods prove the validity and advantage of our system, especially guaranteeing good balance between the interpretability and precision of predictions in HKDP.

Keywords: Hybrid knowledge graph · Pediatric disease prediction system · Naïve Bayes · Multi-label classification

1 Introduction

Various computational models have been used to predict disease based on clinical data [1, 2]. Expert systems based on logic and rules were developed in last century [3]. Recent developments in statistical models provide new opportunities for implementing intelligent disease prediction [4]. There are still many challenges in realizing a practical predictive model. One of key problems is how to build a predictive model from heterogeneous data sources. In particular, human doctors make decisions on multiple

C. Xing et al. (Eds.): ICSH 2016, LNCS 10219, pp. 78–90, 2017.
DOI: 10.1007/978-3-319-59858-1_8

possible diseases based on both clinical experiences and knowledge learned from text books, while most of machine learning models focus on the clinical data which contains just one type of diseases. There is still, to the best of the author's knowledge, few works to build a comprehensive model over heterogeneous data sources for predicting multiple diseases.

The work presented in this paper provides a systematic solution towards this issue. Specifically, we proposed a Hybrid Knowledge graph model based pediatric Disease Prediction system (HKDP) to integrate a Bayesian statistic model with knowledge pieces extracted from clinical data, text book and expert experiences. In the system, a multi-label prediction classifier is designed to predict diseases based on clinical symptom descriptive texts. We compare the proposed predictive models with other classical methods. The results show that the precision rate, recall rate and F-score are all improved.

The organization of this paper is as follows: Sect. 2 provides an overview of related work on disease perdition models. Section 3 describes the whole framework of the proposed system and the hybrid knowledge graph construction. Section 4 focuses on the disease diagnosis model. Section 5 presents the experimental evaluation. Section 6 gives conclusion and future works.

2   Related Work

Recently more and more computational models have been applied in intelligent tasks such as question-answer [5] and topic discovering from e-health data [6]. Disease prediction, as a classical problem of Clinical Decision Support System (CDSS) research [3], is still receiving much more attentions. Current major researches on disease prediction focus on two trends: Bayesian models and Artificial Neural Network (ANN) models.

An early Bayesian model in [7] was investigated to predict the on-set of Alzheimer's disease. [8] has done some research on the suitability of the Gaussian Bayes classifier in determining DR severity level. The Bayesian model was also used in the prediction of heart disease [9, 10]. In [11, 12], two similar heart disease prediction systems based on a naïve Bayes model were proposed respectively, both of which predict the likelihood of patients getting a heart disease, whereas the latter also used a Jelinek-mercer smoothing technique to improve the prediction. In order to compensate for the deficiencies of Bayesian models in heart disease prediction, Nahar has proposed two different improvement methods. One was a feature extraction method based on medical knowledge, which had shown promise in heart disease diagnostics [13]; another was using several rule mining algorithms (Apriori, Predictive Apriori and Tertius) to find association rules in heart disease data which then be applied to a naïve Bayes classifier and had made a favor to identify the key factors behind the disease [14].

Neural network models have been extensively applied in intelligent medication systems. The work can be traced back to 1990s, when artificial neural network began to apply to clinical medicine [15]. In [16], Dawson applied the Bayesian model and Recurrent Neural Networks (RNN) to medical image analysis. Inouye et al. [17] presented a predictive model using admission characteristics which classify delirium in order to help discover potential disease. Recently, significant achievements in deep neural network models provide new opportunities in making more intelligent prediction models based on big data. For example, a diagnostic model based on the Long Short Term Memory (LSTM) model was proposed which established the patient characteristics by identifying the time series and then used the RNN to build the predictive model [18]. This model has a good effect in diagnosing diabetes. On the same time, Google researchers proposed an unsupervised deep feature learning method to extract feature information from Electronic Medical Records (EHR) data and established a better model to predict latent possible diseases [19]. Neural network models are black-box models and are difficult to explain. In order to solve this problem, Zhihua Zhou proposed a C4.5 rule model using artificial neural network to do data preprocessing, which has strong interpretability due to the advantages of rule induction [20].

Most previous work are based on EHR. There is still few work on incorporating heterogeneous data and knowledge that are from both EHR and text books. Moreover, most models are single-disease model, which is not suitable for a real clinical application that will face multiple possible diseases. In this paper, we provide a hybrid knowledge graph model to address these two problems.

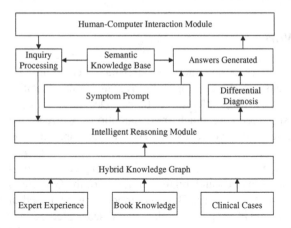

Fig. 1. The system architecture diagram

3   System Architecture

Figure 1 shows the architecture diagram of the proposed system which consists of following models: *The human-computer interaction module* receives input from users and displays the returned results. The *inquiry processing module* is built to process the user input and apply the natural language processing method to identify the relevant feature information from the text of user input. *The answers generation module* generates the output sentences according to the user input and the results from the intelligent reasoning model. *The intelligent reasoning module* conduct reasons over the hybrid knowledge graph according to the information from heterogeneous data sources in expertise knowledge, case base and book knowledge and the module will provide disease prediction results or prompt for user to continue providing more symptoms. ***The symptom prompt module*** use a Latent Dirichlet Allocation (LDA) [21] to analyze the clinical case feature graph and locates the top-k symptoms as the recommendation for users to evaluate. The system also recommends more symptoms with the largest weights according to the previous inputs of users. ***Differential diagnosis module*** combines symptom information entered by the user with the somatoscopy information and uses the diagnostic criteria of the top-*k* most matching diseases to build a final differential diagnosis based on a multiple labeling prediction model that is built based on the hybrid knowledge graph. ***Differential diagnosis module*** is the core module to implement the prediction function in the system. The core methods will be introduced in next sections.

The prediction is based on knowledge extracted from different sources including: ***Expert experience library*** mainly comes from the oral dictation of doctors; ***Semantic Knowledge Base*** containing common symptoms and signs in medicine, and syntax pattern expression rules that are used to parse the natural language text. ***Book Knowledge Base*** contains a large number of entity-relationship information that extracted from a college text book in *Pediatrics*. ***Case database*** contains 1454 raw clinically pediatric cases that come from a hospital. We build a hybrid knowledge graph to integrate knowledge extracted from these heterogeneous data sources for further reasoning.

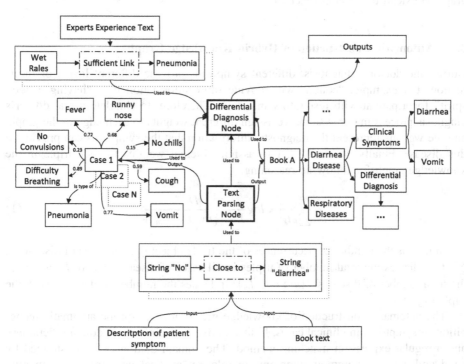

Fig. 2. The structure of the hybrid knowledge graph

3.1   Structure of Hybrid Knowledge Graph

We design a hybrid knowledge graph structure to hold knowledge information from heterogeneous sources. More specifically, we use the hybrid knowledge graph to integrate a statistical model, a rule based model, and a semantic pattern model in one structure so that it can support future extension. The hybrid knowledge graph is a labelled graph consisting of following types of nodes: *disease types, symptom types, syntax objects* and *computational nodes*; Links are of types: *Bayesian priori-probability, sufficient condition, existence positioning relation* and *computer input/output*. Disease types, symptoms and syntax objects are linked by those edges to represent reasoning semantics and natural language parsing semantics. Computational nodes in the graph are processing algorithms that take inputting nodes as arguments and take outputs also as nodes in the graph. Figure 2 shows a basic structure of a hybrid knowledge graph.

For example, the **text parsing** node in Fig. 2 takes a set of semantic parsing links as its input and extracts semantics information from natural language of the text book and user input texts. The output of the **text parsing** node contains multiple entity-relationships that will be integrated into the hybrid knowledge graph. When processing a reasoning task, the **text parsing** node is also invoked to parse relevant texts into semantic structures for further usage. A run-time execution engine is implemented in the **intelligent reasoning module** to hold the hybrid knowledge graph and support the running. In this way, we can dynamically update the hybrid knowledge graph to extend the system function.

3.2   Automatic Construction of Hybrid Knowledge Graph

During the doctor's diagnosis, different symptoms provide different levels of information. For example, "cough" will provide more information than "having a good spirit" for a patient with respiratory infection. Therefore, to simulate a real doctor's diagnosis process in our system, we assign different weights to each edge in the graph, and the weights represent the diagnostic information that the symptoms can provide in this disease. Finally, we use Eq. 1 to assign different weights to each triple in the knowledge graph for follow-up reasoning.

$$\omega_{ij} \frac{t_{ij}}{\sum_k t_{kj}} \times log \frac{|D|}{1 + |\{m : t_i \in d_m\}|} \tag{1}$$

In it, t_{ij} is the number of occurrences of the triple object t_i in all cases of disease d_j, $\sum_k t_{kj}$ indicates the total number of triples in all cases of disease d_j, and $|D|$ indicates the total number of diseases. $|\{m : t_i \in d_m\}|$ indicates the number of diseases with the triple object t_i.

The automatic construction of knowledge graphs focuses on the automatic recognition of symptoms in clinical cases. In this study, we mainly use a domain dictionary and a regular expression matching method. The domain dictionary is constructed by hand and contains common symptoms in relevant medical domains. Subsequently, regular expressions are constructed by this domain dictionary, which is used to identify the symptoms of each clinically pediatric case. Besides, the extraction method based on the domain dictionary and regular expressions are also used to find rules from expert experiences and to parse the text book, and then we mix up all results into the hybrid knowledge graph. In summary, the construction of the disease knowledge graph can be described by the following steps.

1. Use the constructed regular expression to extract the symptoms in the cases.
2. Construct triples with the symptoms.
3. Represent the disease as a set of triples and calculate the number of occurrences of different diseases.
4. Construct graph for each disease, calculate the prior probabilities for symptoms and add the weights to the graph.
5. Find rules from expert experience and parse the text book.
6. Mix up the graph, rules and the knowledge of text book into a hybrid knowledge graph and add edges.

4 Disease Diagnosis Model

Based on the detailed analysis of 1454 clinically pediatric cases, we found that doctors always consider more than one type of diseases when making a diagnose over a case, and rank the diseases according to the likelihood they measure. With this in mind, we model the problem of disease diagnosis as a multi-label classification problem considering labels order. In this section, we propose a hierarchical disease diagnosis model based on a naive Bayesian model, rules as well as book knowledge which have been formalized in the hybrid knowledge graph. Figure 3 shows the block diagram of this hierarchical model. When diagnosing a clinical case, the multi-label classification based on naïve Bayes is used firstly, which predict several diseases with probability, then we use the rule-based and the book-knowledge-based reasoning to filter and fill up possible results.

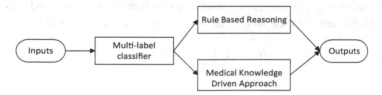

Fig. 3. The block diagram of the hierarchical model

4.1 Naïve Bayes Based Multi-label Classifier

Naive Bayes Classifier
Naïve Bayes is a classical statistical classifier which assumes no dependency between attributes. It works as follows:

Let the input space $x \subseteq R^n$ be a set of n-dimensional vectors, and the output space $y = \{c_1, c_2, \ldots, c_i\}$ be a set of class labels. The input is a feature vector $x \in x$, and the output is a class label $y \in y$. X is a random variable defined in the input space and Y is a random variable defined in the output space. $P(X, Y)$ is the joint probability distribution of X and Y. The training dataset $T = \{(x_1, y_1), (x_2, y_2), \ldots, (x_N, y_N)\}$ is generated by an independent identical distribution $P(X, Y)$. A Naïve Bayesian model learns the joint probability distribution $P(X, Y)$ by training over the known dataset. Given the input x, the posterior probability distribution is calculated by the learned model, and the label with the largest posterior probability is regarded as the outputs.

$$y = f(x) = argmax_{c_i} \frac{P(Y = c_i) \prod_{j=1}^{n} P(X^{(j)} = x^{(j)} | Y = c_i)}{\sum_i P(Y = c_i) \prod_{j=1}^{n} P(X^{(j)} = x^{(j)} | Y = c_i)} \tag{2}$$

Note that the denominator in the above equation is the same for all c_i, so the final formula is

$$y = argmax_{c_i} P(Y = c_i) \prod_{j=1}^{n} P\left(X^{(j)} = x^{(j)} | Y = c_i\right) \tag{3}$$

$$argmax_{c_i} P(Y = c_i) \prod_{j=1}^{n} \omega_{ij} \tag{4}$$

where ω_{ij} is the weight of tripe in disease c_i in the hybrid knowledge graph.

Multi-label Classifier

The classic Naïve Bayes classification algorithm is effective for single-label samples, however, in our clinical cases, one sample always contains multiple class labels, which makes it tricky for us to directly use. To solve this problem, we adopted a one-vs-all strategy [22] which learns $|L|$ naïve Bayes binary classifiers $H_l : X \rightarrow \{l, \neg l\}$, one for each different disease label l in L, where L is the number of labels of diseases. The original training data set is transformed into $|L|$ data sets D_l that contain all examples of the original training data set, labelled as l if the labels of the original example contained l and as $\neg l$ otherwise. For the classification of a new instance x this method outputs as a set of labels the union of the labels that are output by the $|L|$ Bayes classifier:

$$H(x) = \bigcup_{l \in L} \{l\} : H_l(x) = l \tag{5}$$

Next, we focus on the determination of the order and number of labels. Here we proposed a mechanism called Average Interval Filtering for dynamically adjusting the number of predicted labels. We rank the labels reversely by their posterior probability, and then extract the top k labels, calculate the average interval between them.

Lastly, we traverse the ranked labels from the second label to the kth label one by one in a way that the current label will be added into the final labels set if the absolute value of the posterior probability of current label and its previous one is smaller than

Table 1. ALGORITHM A: average_interval_filtering

	ALGORITHM A: *average_interval_filtering (p)*
	RETURNS: The prediction set of labels *label_sets*
1	$avg\_inv = \mathrm{abs}(p(l_1)\text{-}p(l_k))$;
2	*label_sets* = $\{l_1\}$;
3	For l in $[l_2\text{:}l_k]$
4	if $\mathrm{abs}(p(l) - p(prev(l))) <= avg\_inv$:
5	*label_sets*.add(l)
6	else:
7	break
	return *label_sets*

the average interval otherwise the traversing is stopped. Due to the fact that a sample must have at least one label, the label with the largest posterior probability will be added into the labels set firstly with no doubt, Table 1 shows the pseudo code.

4.2 Rule Based Reasoning

In the above work, we have formalized the experience of domain experts into the form of {*IF...THEN...*} rules in the hybrid knowledge graph. There are two different kinds of rules in the hybrid knowledge graph, namely, the sufficient condition rule and the necessary condition rule. The sufficient condition rules can be used straightforwardly with the form of {*IF* $s_1, s_2...THEN d_1, d_2...$}. With the symptoms that we extract, we try to match them using the prefixes in the sufficient condition rules. If the match is successful, the suffixes of the sufficient condition rules which are also the disease labels will be directly added into the set of sample labels. The difference we make use of the necessary condition rules with the form of {*IF* d_1 *THEN* $s_1, s_2...$} is that the labels we predicted from the above classifier will be re-filtered by the necessary condition rules. Given the label l in the predicted labels set, we will check whether the symptoms of patients meet the suffixes of the necessary condition rule. If not, the label l will be eliminated from the predicted labels set.

4.3 Medical Knowledge Driven Approach

In order to further improve the accuracy of the predicted results, we finally use the knowledge of medical books driven approach to identify the disease label in the predicted labels set. The knowledge of medical books has been formalized to XML format, in which the ⟨differential diagnosis⟩ tag records the conditions for the final diagnosis of a disease. Therefore, we will compare the symptoms that we extract from clinical case with the conditions for diagnosis of each disease label in predicted labels set, and the disease label will be one of the eventually outputs if the difference is within an acceptable range, otherwise the disease label is removed.

5 Evaluation

In this section, we introduce the evaluation metrics used in the system. Compared with the traditional single-label classification, multi-label classification usually requires more complex evaluation metrics. In our system, we use precision, recall and F-score [22]. Let D is a data set containing D multi-label samples which can be expressed as $(x_i, y_i), i = 1 \ldots |D|$. L is the set of disease tags. H is a multi-label classifier, $Z_i = H(x_i)$ is the set of labels predicted by sample x_i.

The precision is the ratio of all correct results in the returned results with all returned results.

$$Precision(H, D) = \frac{1}{|D|} \sum_{i=1}^{|D|} \frac{|Y_i \bigcap Z_i|}{|Z_i|} \tag{6}$$

The recall is expressed as the ratio of all correct results in the returned results with all the original correct results.

$$Recall(H, D) = \frac{1}{|D|} \sum_{i=1}^{|D|} \frac{|Y_i \bigcap Z_i|}{|Y_i|} \tag{7}$$

Accuracy and recall have different emphases, and F-score can be used to balance them. F-value is defined as follows.

$$F(H, D) = \frac{2 * Precision(H, D) * Recall(H, D)}{Precision(H, D) + Recall(H, D)} \tag{8}$$

5.1 Experiment Results

The dataset contains 1454 clinically pediatric cases in which each sample contains several disease labels and the total number of types of diseases is 71. Because of the imbalance distribution of disease labels in the raw dataset, we totally conducted 5 experiments for each test model and each time we randomly selected 80% samples for training and prediction. Here, we mainly do two groups of contrast experiments. First, we compared our model with the traditional Bayes based multi-label classification model which uses the TF-IDF method for feature extraction. Table 2 presents the values of the evaluation parameters (precision, recall, F-score) of the predictive models. We can see that the average of precision value, recall value and F-score of HKDP are all about 12% larger than TFIDF-NB. Figure 4 illustrates the trends of precision value, recall value and F-score of HKDP and TFIDF-NB in 5 experiments.

Second, we applied the method of feature extraction we used for constructing the hybrid knowledge graph automatically to the classical classifier including SVM, KNN and Logistic Regression. As we can see in Table 3, HKDP also performs better than all other classifiers. The reason is that the book knowledge and expert rules play a significant role in identifying and replenishing the diseases. Besides, the trend graph in

Table 2. The precision value, recall value and F-score of HKDP and TFIDF-NB

Exp.	HKDP			TFIDF-NB		
	Precision	Recall	F-score	Precision	Recall	Recall
1	0.7597	0.7217	0.7245	0.6571	0.6076	0.6066
2	0.7494	0.7170	0.7163	0.6254	0.5683	0.5749
3	0.7627	0.7212	0.7255	0.6399	0.5946	0.5935
4	0.7621	0.7295	0.7300	0.6332	0.5704	0.5784
5	0.7696	0.7210	0.7274	0.6572	0.6052	0.6061
avg	0.7607	0.7221	0.7247	0.6426	0.5892	0.5919

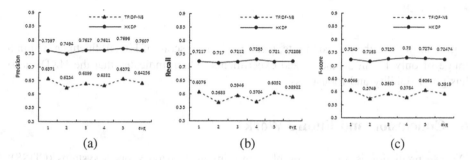

(a)   (b)   (c)

Fig. 4. The trend graphs of precision value (a), recall value (b) and F-score (c) of HKDP and TFIDF-NB

Table 3. The precision value, recall value and F-score of HKDP, SVM, KNN and LR

Exp.	HKDP			SVM		
	Precision	Recall	F-score	Precision	Recall	F-score
1	0.7597	0.7217	0.7245	0.6260	0.5877	0.5855
2	0.7494	0.7170	0.7163	0.5848	0.5651	0.5543
3	0.7627	0.7212	0.7255	0.6352	0.5873	0.5896
4	0.7621	0.7295	0.7300	0.6441	0.5992	0.5993
5	0.7696	0.7210	0.7274	0.6344	0.5896	0.5890
avg	0.7607	0.7221	0.7247	0.6249	0.5858	0.5835
Exp.	KNN			LR		
	Precision	Recall	F-score	Precision	Recall	F-score
1	0.6505	0.5624	0.5805	0.6189	0.5585	0.5657
2	0.6222	0.5545	0.5648	0.6182	0.5525	0.5608
3	0.6298	0.5516	0.5658	0.6154	0.5514	0.5606
4	0.5980	0.5381	0.5464	0.6334	0.5701	0.5783
5	0.5989	0.5290	0.5410	0.6260	0.5643	0.5703
avg	0.6199	0.5471	0.5597	0.6224	0.5594	0.5671

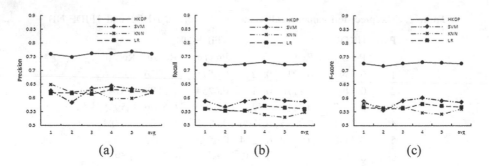

(a)   (b)   (c)

Fig. 5. The trend graphs of precision value (a), recall value (b) and F-score (c) of HKDP, SVM, KNN and LR

Fig. 5 shows that the precision rate, recall rate and F-score of HKDP fluctuate within a range of only 1% in 5 randomized experiments, which indicates that the HKDP also has good stability and robustness.

6   Conclusion and Future Work

Disease prediction is a classic problem in clinical decision support systems (CDSS). One of the new problems is how to improve the accuracy of prediction with multiple heterogeneous data sources. In this paper, we presented a hybrid knowledge graph, which is used to integrate the clinically pediatric cases, classically professional pediatrics textbooks as well as clinical experiences of pediatric doctors, and the automatic construction method of this hybrid knowledge graph. Based on this graph, we built a disease prediction system which provides a multi-label classifier with label filtering. The system parses the descriptive text of patent's symptoms and uses the knowledge in hybrid knowledge graph for intelligent reasoning and returns the predicted diseases results for patients finally. We conducted experiments on the 1454 clinical cases and the results show that HKDP has better prediction precision, recall and F-score than SVM, KNN, and LR, and has good interpretability at the same time.

In the future work, we will further expand the hybrid knowledge graph, introducing and studying the cognitive simulation model, so that the knowledge graph can simulate the thinking and evaluation process of medical diagnosis of doctors, and thus has better extensibility and self-explanation. Furthermore, we will apply our methods to the Traditional Chinese Medicine(TCM), in order to build a hybrid knowledge graph over TCM data for assisting diagnosis making of TCM.

Acknowledgments. This work was supported by the Networked Operating System for Cloud Computing (Grant No. 2016YFB1000505) and the Special Program for Applied Research on Super Computation of the NSFC-Guangdong Joint Fund (the second phase). Thanks Zongbo Zhang, Han Li and Dongxue Huo for some preliminary work.

References

1. Alshayea, Q.: Artificial neural networks in medical diagnosis. Int. J. Comput. Sci. Issues **96**, 197–228 (2011)
2. Lin, D., Vasilakos, A.V., Tang, Y., Yao, Y.: Neural networks for computer-aided diagnosis in medicine: a review. Neurocomputing **216**, 700–708 (2016)
3. Shortliffe, E.H.: MYCIN: Computer-Based Medical Consultations. Elsevier, New York (1976)
4. Prema, S., Umamaheswari, P.: Multitude classifier using rough set jelinek mercer Naïve Bayes for disease diagnosis. Circ. Syst. **07**, 701–708 (2016)
5. Zhang, Y., Zhang, Y., Yin, Y., Xu, J., Xing, C., Chen, H.: Chronic disease related entity extraction in online chinese question and answer services. In: Zheng, X., Zeng, D.D., Chen, H., Leischow, Scott J. (eds.) ICSH 2015. LNCS, vol. 9545, pp. 55–67. Springer, Cham (2016). doi:10.1007/978-3-319-29175-8_6
6. Chen, X., Zhang, Y., Xu, J., Xing, C., Chen, H.: Deep learning based topic identification and categorization: mining diabetes-related topics on Chinese health websites. In: Navathe, Shamkant B., Wu, W., Shekhar, S., Du, X., Wang, X.S., Xiong, H. (eds.) DASFAA 2016. LNCS, vol. 9642, pp. 481–500. Springer, Cham (2016). doi:10.1007/978-3-319-32025-0_30
7. Prince, M.J.: Predicting the onset of Alzheimer's disease using Bayes' theorem. Am. J. Epidemiol. **143**, 301–308 (1996)
8. Hani, A.F.M., Nugroho, H.A., Nugroho, H.: Gaussian Bayes classifier for medical diagnosis and grading: Application to diabetic retinopathy. In: Biomedical Engineering and Sciences, pp. 52–56 (2010)
9. Subbalakshmi, G., Ramesh, K., Rao, M.C.: Decision support in heart disease prediction system using Naive Bayes. Indian J. Comput. Sci. Eng. **2**, 170–176 (2011)
10. Dangare, C.S., Apte, S.S.: Improved study of heart disease prediction system using data mining classification techniques. Int. J. Comput. Appl. **47**, 44–48 (2012)
11. Patil, A.P., Bhosale, A.P., Ambre, G.: Intelligent Heart Disease Prediction System using Naive Bayes Classifier. Int. J. Adv. Innov. Res. (2013)
12. Patil, M.R.R.: Heart disease prediction system using Naive Bayes and Jelinek-mercer smoothing. Int. J. Adv. Res. Comput. Commun. Eng. **3**, 6787–6792 (2014)
13. Nahar, J., Imam, T., Tickle, K.S., Chen, Y.P.P.: Computational intelligence for heart disease diagnosis: a medical knowledge driven approach. Expert Syst. Appl. **40**, 96–104 (2013)
14. Nahar, J., Imam, T., Tickle, K.S., Chen, Y.P.P.: Association rule mining to detect factors which contribute to heart disease in males and females. Expert Syst. Appl. **40**, 1086–1093 (2013)
15. Baxt, W.G.: Application of artificial neural networks to clinical medicine. Lancet **346**, 1135–1138 (1995)
16. Dawson, A., Austin Jr., R., Weinberg, D.: Nuclear grading of breast carcinoma by image analysis. Classification by multivariate and neural network analysis. Am. J. Clin. Pathol. **95**, S29–S37 (1991)
17. Inouye, S.K., Viscoli, C.M., Horwitz, R.I., Hurst, L.D., Tinetti, M.E.: A predictive model for delirium in hospitalized elderly medical patients based on admission characteristics. Ann. Internal Med. **119**, 474–481 (1993)
18. Lipton, Z.C., Kale, D.C., Elkan, C., Wetzell, R.: Learning to diagnose with LSTM recurrent neural networks. Comput. Sci. (2015)
19. Miotto, R., Li, L., Kidd, B.A., Dudley, J.T.: Deep patient: an unsupervised representation to predict the future of patients from the electronic health records. Sci. Rep. **6** (2016)

20. Zhou, Z.-H., Jiang, Y.: Medical diagnosis with C4. 5 rule preceded by artificial neural network ensemble. IEEE Trans. Inf Technol. Biomed. **7**, 37–42 (2003)
21. Blei, D.M., Ng, A.Y., Jordan, M.I.: Latent dirichlet allocation. J. Mach. Learn. Res. **3**, 993–1022 (2003)
22. Tsoumakas, G., Katakis, I.: Multi-label Classification: An Overview. Department of Informatics, Aristotle University of Thessaloniki, Greece (2006)

Research on the Smartphone Based eHealth Systems for Strengthing Healthcare Organization

Uzair Aslam Bhatti[1,2(✉)], Mengxing Huang[1,2(✉)], Yu Zhang[2], and Wenlong Feng[2]

[1] State Key Laboratory of Marine Resource Utilization in South China Sea, Hainan University, Haikou 570228, China
uzairaslambhatti@hotmail.com, huangmx09@163.com
[2] College of Information Science and Technology, Hainan University, Haikou, Hainan, China

Abstract. Data collection is the primary prerequisite in health sector whenever an organization craving to fortify and improve its health system. In early phases of expansion and advancement in health sector data collection was paper based, which repel in analysis on daily basis because of gigantic data is available on daily basis and manual calculation and analysis is not possible. So for removing that encumbrance of analysis the manual paper based data collection is then entered into health MIS system which help a lot in analysis purpose. But that was not as faster in development and analysis phase which help analytical analysis of trends of Diseases, Equipment's, Vaccines and punctuality of Staff of health organization also the problems of developing countries cannot afford MIS systems in rural areas thus there is a need of solution to tackle information collection and timely analysis with submissions. In this paper, the concept of Smartphone based healthcare strengthen system is shared which will reduce the burden of data collection also speed up the process of data analysis and reduce the burden. Paper work can be reduce and no need of punching the data in some health MIS system. Smart phone application also gives the concept how the monitoring staff performance and healthcare organization regularity and punctuality can be analyzed. Complete this system is developed using open source frameworks and developed application is used on smartphones having android OS. Project is implemented in Pakistan and is being used successfully in 24 districts and this project brought a drastic change in the organization in the decision making process and also for improving the poor healthcare indicators.

Keywords: Big data · Healthcare MIS · Smart health · Monitoring health system

1 Introduction

The qualitative data analysis is yet the biggest issue in developing countries as compared to the developed countries because of the lake of availability of quality resources which help out in timely analysis of the data. Lack of adequate tools to measure research use remains the missing link for a meaningful evaluation of any strategy which aims at increasing the influence of research results. Since about 1990, many developing and transition countries have undertaken market-oriented reforms in their electric power

© Springer International Publishing AG 2017
C. Xing et al. (Eds.): ICSH 2016, LNCS 10219, pp. 91–101, 2017.
DOI: 10.1007/978-3-319-59858-1_9

sectors. Despite the widespread adoption of a standard policy model, reform processes and outcomes have often failed to meet expectations (Electricity Market Reform and Deregulation, Volume 31, Issues 6–7, May–June 2006, Pages 815–844). Thus there is the need of the system which helps out the timely submission of data in rural areas so that data analysis can be taken place which will not be depend over the things like electricity, computers and storages over rural areas. This paper presents the smart phone solution for purpose of data collection with many benefits to tackle out above mentioned issues. It helps saving of computer as data is collected over smart phone, secondly it not required much electricity as battery backup of mobile phone is too much for job hours and also smart phones are easily to carry from one health center to other health center. The collected data can be sent to centralized server once the internet connectivity is available. The paper research is analyzed in a country Pakistan where qualitative data collection is yet the biggest issue and it is lagged behind its neighbors and many other low income countries in relation to health indicators. This is mainly due to low spending on social sectors and poor management of health services. The progress in achievement of Millennium Development Goals (MDGs) such as reducing infant mortality rate to 40, under 5 mortality rates to 52 and maternal mortality to 140 by 2015 seems illusory (Economic Survey of Pakistan (ESP) 2012–2013: p. 147). Spending on Health through public and private sectors is extremely low and 0.35% of GDP (ESP 2012–2013: p. 147). The population growth rate in 2008 (www.google.com/publicdata) was estimated at 2.14% per annum which is high. The total fertility rate is 3.8 (Pakistan Demographic and Health survey (PDHS) 2002–13: p. 11) as compared to 5.4 at the beginning of 1990s (PDHS 1990/91). The contraceptive prevalence rate is estimated to be as low as 35% (PDHS 2012–13: p. 23). Maternal Mortality Ratio (MMR) per 100,000 live births is pitched at 276. The Infant Mortality Rate (IMR) was 78/1000 live births for the period 2002–06 compared to 91 per 1000 in 1986–89 (Pakistan Integrated Household Survey 2006/07). All in all, according to a survey Pakistan has failed to achieve, 'Health for All' due to lack of transparency, inadequate public funding, and poor governance resulting in poor quality of public services. The most basic issue identified by the Government is that despite injection of billions of rupees, doctor and medicines are not available to the poor people in rural areas of Sindh. The main issues at the FLCFs (First Level Healthcare Facilities) have been identified & include: (i). Absence of Staff (About 35% reported across Bangladesh, Ecuador, India, Indonesia, Peru and Uganda reported in Chaudhry et al. 2006). (ii). Non availability of medicine (iii). Poor vaccination. (iv). Illegal occupation of HFs (Health Facilities) by local Feudal. (vi). Poor availability of family planning material and others. In order to improve the delivery of services, Government of Sindh has contracted out the management of Basic Health Units (BHUs) to a Non Profit Organization-PHC Sindh in 2007 along with existing budget, in order to improve delivery of health services. PHC Sindh-an organization registered under Companies Ordinance 1979, has introduced the use of smart phone as a measure of control to collect reports relating to various Primary Health Care indicators. In this paper, we will analyse the importance of use of smart phone as a measure of control, its significance and benefits accrued to the organization in the context of management theories. This is an innovative idea and no such Information and Communication Technology (ICT) intervention introduced before in the Province of Sindh especially in the health

Sector. This evaluation will add value to the literature, as well present a precedent for a developing countries to replicate and adopt in their respective health systems.

In this paper, Sect. 2 will review the Background of ICT in health sector. Section 3, Research methodology with approach, Sect. 4, Implementation and Evaluation and in the last section we will present conclusion and recommendations.

2 Background

2.1 Control and Management

The concept of control is in an organization is located within different theoretical perspectives, including cybernetics theory, labor process, neo-institutionalism and structuration theories as well as post structuralism approaches (Klecun et al. 2014, p. 3). In this paper we will analyze work level or field work, which is a Micro level as Macro level usually involve global perspectives. The research on control has discussed with respect to identity/power, resistance, materiality and context (Delbridge and Ezzamel 2005, p. 604). However in management literature it addresses managerial concerns of controlling workforce, coordination of activities and achieving technical efficiency (Flamholtz et al. 1985). Different perspectives (Structural, administrative & Psychological) on control, emphasize different mechanisms of control. The controls are depicted in the literature as enabling i.e. they facilitate coordinated action and constraining that they constrain the outcomes of the individuals. Furthermore, control mechanisms are interwoven with trust relationships especially in a professional work. Since, the healthcare workers are seen as Professionals & knowledge workers as they managed knowledge itself & expert power and trust and they can be easily adjusted in data processing environments therefore, they can facilitate work, which is also visible and auditable.

2.2 Information and Communication Technology (ICT) and Monitoring in Health Sector

There are different views in the literature (ICT) about the effect of the ICT on managerial processes as well as, on people. The majority view in the literature considers ICT as enabling tool and tends to increase both workforce and process controls (Orlkowski 1991). Although, it is accepted that people have agency to resist such controls (Alvarez 2008; Ball and Wilson 2000; Doolin 1998). ICT may facilitate surveillance and accumulation of knowledge about people and groups through data collection, and warehousing, data mining analysis, dashboards and benchmarking thus creating filed of visibility (Klecun et al. 2014, p. 5). According to Doolin 1998, those who are aware that they are subject of field of visibility then they exercise self discipline. One of the argue is that "IT is supplanting hierarchy's role in coordinating and controlling activities. As a result it has become one of the threads from which the fabric of organization is now woven." Information system such as those targeted at recording, monitoring and evaluating activities, facilitates various types of control by making individuals in organizations "both calculable and calculating with respect to their own actions". Kallinikos and Hasselbladh (2009, p. 263) suggest that ICT should be understood as bringing together regimes of work and regimes of control. Hence, computation changes both the content & object of the work and regimes of control. The classification of the different perspective on control, role assigned to ICT and topic discussed in literature has been classified by Klecun et al. 2014, p. 7 and is given in Appendix 5.

This paper is relating to the evaluation in the context of managerial control to improve technical efficiency and will evaluate the impact of ICT on the motivation of the ICT and outcomes achieved.

2.3   Why Smart Phone Monitoring System

In order to establish a better control firms have to develop smart monitoring systems, PHC management has introduced smart phone monitoring system. The PHC monitoring staff, are issued an android phones and imparted training on the use of a software installed on each Phone. These smart phones enable the monitors, to upload the results of their assigned visit to a dashboard, which instantly compile results on a centralized server to generate instant output. This aggregated information captured by the most recent visit to a central database using General Packet Radio Service (GPRS) in real time. Data are then presented in a summary of tables, charts and graphs and accordingly action is taken at different levels of management (Fig. 1).

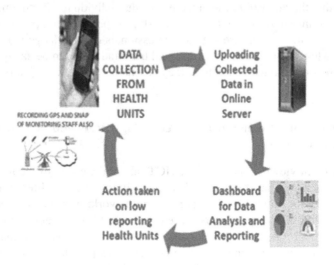

Fig. 1. Basic framwork of mobile smart phone monitoring implementation

3   Research Methodology and Approach

3.1   Overview of Methodology

This observational descriptive study has been carried out in one of the province of Pakistan-Sindh. PHC Sindh is using smart phones in twenty four districts under its management. The two districts out of the six using smart phone monitoring, namely Hyderabad and Sukkur has been selected on random basis for the present study.

3.2   Source of Data

The data has been collected through both qualitative and quantitative sources. A Research questionnaire was developed for interview of the officers of PHC involved in the use of smart phone monitoring. The interview was carried out from the officers. The list of interview includes the software engineers who are involved in the inputs, process and out puts/outcome indicators of smart phone monitoring system. The existing record and reports sent by the monitors were also collected, evaluated/observed at provincial level by researcher and recorded on the designed formats.

3.3   Data Analysis

Data is collected via mobile application from different hospitals while that data is sent to the centralized server for the purpose of the report generation and analysis. Centralized server is having PHP as front end and for backend database we have used MySQL. Server is using Ubuntu as OS with ODK (Open Data Kit) server installed. All the above tools for analysis and compilation are open source and supports native soft wares.

4   Implementation and Evaluation

The entire monitoring staffs are found trained in the use of smart phone monitoring system. All of them were found in possession of and comfortable, in use of smart phone as a monitoring tool. They think that it is economical to use smart phone. Besides, uses of ICT save their time. All (100%) interviewee confirmed to send collected data on daily basis. The data is available to be utilized at district, regional and provincial offices at the close of hours on daily basis.

There is large number of Primary Healthcare indicators, which could be monitored through smart Phone. However, after in-house discussion, PHC has finalized to collect initially data relating to the areas mentioned in Table 1 above. On a query as to why only these indicators? PHC management informed that they used to produce monthly DHIS reports to generate policy actions. However, these indicators are chosen to see the progress in these indicators on daily basis which include timely accurate and actionable information.

Table 1. Type & nature of the data collected

Data collected	Total respondents	Responded			
		Yes		No	
Facility utilization data	10	10	100%	0	0%
Data accuracy	10	0	0%	10	100%
MCH Services	10	10	100%	0	0%
HR regularity punctuality	10	10	100%	0	0%
Essential medicine use. Wastage, balance and stock out status	10	10	100%	0	0%
Vaccine use. Wastage, balance and stock out status	10	10	100%	0	0%
Family planning commodities use, wastage, balance and stock out status	10	10	100%	0	0%
Tracking of monitors	10	10	100%	0	0%

Apart from interviews, outcome data and actionable evidence has been collected from the Head office. It has been informed that PHC is working on the following outcome indicators. The objective is to take action on the reports, at all levels, on daily basis. The following reports are produced by PHC, which are analyzed as under:-

4.1 Absenteeism of Medical and Paramedical Staff

PHC Sindh has two categories of medical and paramedical staff working at about 1135 HFs. First, called as 'government staff'- those were recruited by the government under their terms and conditions. They were present at the respective HFs prior to the management take over by PHC. The staffs is given service protection at the time of signing of the agreement. It is the reason that their hire and fire vests with government. In case of their absence, PHC management will send reports to the Health department for initiation of disciplinary action. The second category is, "PHC staff ", who is appointed by PHC

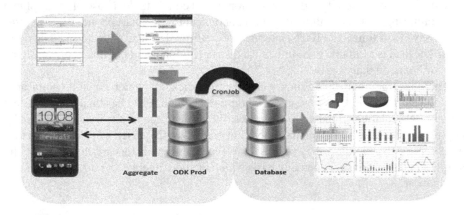

Fig. 2. Framework of mobile application

on a contract basis and their hire and fire vests with PHC. The Fig. 2 shows that staff absenteeism is increased in August as compared to June, 2016. This may be due to a coordinated, well spread out visits and due to the easy collection of data through smart phone. PHC has issued number of letters to the Health department for taking disciplinary action against the absentee government staff.

Habitual Absentees: The software also provides report about the staff with their names and place of posting as well their frequency of absence in a month or comparative in two months. The Fig. 3 mentions about the staff, found repeatedly absent during the month of June to August, 2016 in the two districts.

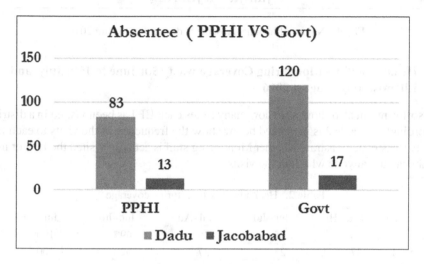

Fig. 3. No of Absentee staff- PHC VS Govt., June to August 2016

4.2 Monitoring of the Monitors

PHC HFs are spread across in the rural areas of the whole Province therefore these are very thinly spread around, geographically. The use of smart phone has resolved their issue of report collection as well as to check the activities of the monitoring staff called as Monitoring of the Monitors. The smart phone allows PHC management at all levels to check whether monitoring staff has actually visited the HF or not through GPRS location system. The monitoring staffs is also required to send pictures of their visit through smart phone as well of the entire staff who is available at the time of visit in the form of group photo. Following Fig. 4 gives the location of the staff vs location of Health Facility.

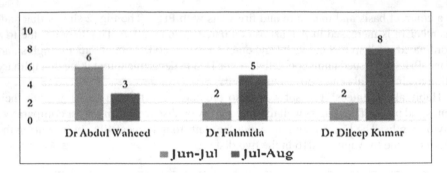

Fig. 4. Names of habitual Absentees during Jun to Aug 2016

4.3 Health Facilities Monitoring Coverage w.e.f 15th June to 15th July, and Likewise July–August 2016

The software can also show as to how many times each HF has been visited in a district. Accordingly, a Table 2 is presented below show the frequency of the visits to each HF. This can easily demonstrate whether Monitoring staff is actually visited the HFs or not? IT can capture anyone who fain the visits.

Table 2. Health facility monitoring coverage

HF coverage	Total HF	Jun–Jul	Jul–Aug	Jun–Jul	Jul–Aug
Dadu	36	25	36	69%	100%
Jacobabad	37	23	37	62%	100%

4.4 Performance of Monitoring Staff

PHC Sindh appoints staff monitoring as well as medical and paramedical staff on a contract basis for a period of six months. The contracts are renewed on the performance every six months by a committee. Therefore, Table 2 mentions the performance of each monitoring staff against the targeted visits. They are issued Memos about the lapses in their achievements (Table 3).

Table 3. Performance of staff

District	DM VISITS			EME			SO		
	Target	Achieved	%	Target	Achieved	%	Target	Achieved	%
Dadu	34	10	29%	60	17	25%	96	75	78%
Jacobabad	34	43	126%	60	15	25%	96	87	91%

4.5 Availability of Functional Equipments

The availability and functionality of essential equipment's has a strong bearing on the quality of services. Figure 5 shows the availability of equipment's through filed re-ports which is not 100% and needs attention of the man-agement of PHC (Fig. 6).

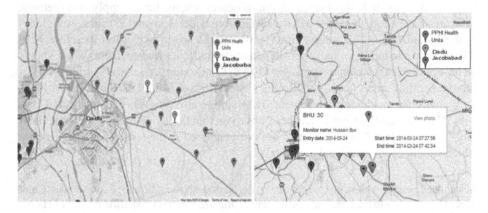

Fig. 5. Location of hospitals and monitoring staff

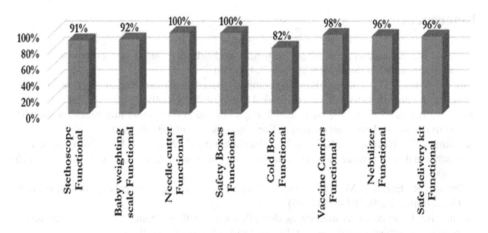

Fig. 6. Availability of equipments

5   Conclusion and Recommendations

This study brought in to a lime light a very innovative idea of the use of ICT as a control in health sector. It has also highlighted as how can technology make things easier, cost effective and saves time of the management. It creates evidence which cannot be denied and this is ideal way to address a big issue of absenteeism, HR management and admin-istration, collecting information, identifying is-sues of supply chain management is a very cost effective and timely manner. However, it is important to caution that it is introduced very recently in PHC therefore findings cannot be generalized immediately however despite the time constraint, this study has a set a platform for fur-there research at a large scale on the subject. This study has identified some of the problems as well, which are of administrative nature and some relate to the software which should be resolved by the management of the PHC. It is also very important that follow up or action is taken on issues such as government staff absenteeism, medicine supply management, equipment's non functionality so that a sustainable effect is created to achieve efficiency in the organization. This intervention is also found worth expansion therefore PHC should now expand it to the other departments under its management. They should include data accuracy monitoring as per LQAS (Lot Quality Assurance Sampling). They should also link smart phone monitoring system with existing DHIS and ERP system for the vaccine, medicine management. They should also cross check smart phone data with DHIS and ERP system IT has been observed that family planning data is regularly sent by the field staff but the reports are not generated at the level of the head office, which should be analyzed and action taken.

Acknowledgment. This work is supported by the National Natural Science Foundation of China under Grant No. 61462022, the Enterprises-universities-researches Integration Project of Hainan under Grant No. cxy20150025.

References

Alvarez, R.: Examining technology, structure and identity during an enterprise system implementation. Inf. Syst. J. **18**(2), 203–224 (2008)

Ball, K., Wilson, D.C.: Power, control and computer-based performance monitoring: repertoires, resistance and subjectivities. Organ. Stud. **21**(3), 539–565 (2000)

Banerjee, A., Duflo, E., Glennerster, R.: Putting a band-aid on a corpse: incentives for users in the Indian public healthcare system. J. Eur. Econ. Assoc. **6**(2–3), 487–500 (2008)

Chaudhury, N., Hammer, J., Kremer, M., Muralidharan, K., Rogers, F.H.: Missing in action: teacher and health worker absence in developing countries. J. Econ. Perspect. **20**(1), 91–116 (2006)

Deibridge, R., Ezzamel, M.: The strength of difference: contemporary conceptions of control. Organization **12**(5), 603–618 (2005)

Doolin, B.: Information technology as disciplinary technology: being critical in interpretive research on information systems. J. Inf. Technol. **13**, 301–311 (1998)

Klecun, E., Cornford, T., Ficociello, M.: ICT and control in healthcare work. Unpublished, London School of Economics (2014)

Flamholtz, E.G., Das, T., Tsui, A.S.: Toward an integrative framework of organizational control. Account. Organ. Soc. **10**(1), 35–50 (1985)

Federal Bureau of Statistics, Statistics Division. Pakistan Integrated Household Survey, 2006–7. Government of Pakistan (2007)

Finance Division: Pakistan Economic Survey of Pakistan 2012–13, Islamabad, Pakistan (2012–13). http://www.finance.gov.pk/survey/survey.htm. Accessed 17 July 2014

Kallinikos, J., Hasselbladh, H.: Work, control and computation: rethinking the legacy of neo-institutionalism. Res. Soc. Organ. (annual) **27**, 241–267 (2009)

National Institute of Population Studies and Macro International Inc: Pakistan Demographic and Health Survey 2012–13. National Institute of Population Studies and Macro International Inc, Islamabad (2012)

National Institute of Population Studies and Macro International Inc.: Pakistan Demographic and Health Survey 1990–91. National Institute of Population Studies and Macro International Inc, Islamabad (1991)

Performance of Finger-Vein Features as a Human Health Indicator

Shilei Liu[✉], He Zheng, Gaoxiong Xu, Liao Ni, Yi Zhang, and Wenxin Li

Institute of Network Computing and Information Systems,
Department of Electronic Engineering and Computer Science,
Peking University, Beijing, China
{cs_lsl,zhenghe,xgx,niliao,zhangyi30.happy,lwx}@pku.edu.cn

Abstract. Biometric features of humans, which include behavioral features and biological features, have two main popular application areas: 1. Biomedical application as in human disease diagnosis and health monitoring; 2. Security application as in identity authentication.

Nowadays, biometric features have great, sometimes even better, performance in certain medical diagnosis areas in comparison to modern medical system, such as heart beats, human breath, tongue image, pulse signal, etc. By using biometric features of human body, biomedical techniques own inherent superiority over traditional medical system on accuracy, speed, sanitation, maintenance and security.

Finger-vein authentication research has been rising since 2003, and has soon become one of the most popular biometric authentication techniques. However, given its inherent advantage as a human feature and great performance in security area, yet by far little has been revealed about whether finger-vein can be used as a human health indicator. In this paper, we discuss what does it take to become a valid health indicator and proceed detailed evaluation on finger-vein features as one. The result shows finger-vein feature is a potential effective indicator for disease early detection and further real-time monitoring on physical condition of human body.

Keywords: Biometric features · Biomedical area · Security area · Finger-vein · Health indicator

1 Introduction

The concept of biometric features consists of two parts: 1. Behavioral features, such as handwriting, voice, gait, etc.; 2. Biological features such as fingerprint, face, iris, finger-vein, etc. Ever since early era of human history, biometric features have played important roles in human life, which can be approximately categorized into two main aspects: Security and Biomedical.

As for security, people determine one's identity based on its appearance and behavior. [1, 3] Nowadays, after years of research, biometric identification techniques using a variety of biometric features are able to automatically determine person's identity at great speed and accuracy. Due to the needs of security usage, this group of biometric

© Springer International Publishing AG 2017
C. Xing et al. (Eds.): ICSH 2016, LNCS 10219, pp. 102–108, 2017.
DOI: 10.1007/978-3-319-59858-1_10

feature shares some good features which includes: 1. Easy to acquire; 2. Zero damage; 3. Immediate results; 4. Low economic cost.

For Biomedical area, there are another group of biometric features that have been proved capable of aiding diseases diagnosis and health conditions monitoring. For example, popular usage of biometric features includes heartbeats pattern (ECG), organ scanning (CT, ultrasonic, MRI), body fluid (blood, urine) analysis, etc. Considering human body is a very complicated and precise system, traditional medical techniques usually suffering from three main problems: 1. high cost on acquisition equipment; 2. patients' unpleasant acquiring experience; 3. longtime of waiting for results.

What if we can use biometric features which are already in security area and apply them to biomedical usage? That way we can take advantage of the inherent good quality and solve the three problems mentioned above.

In fact, researchers have already achieved some goals on this. For example, pulse signal, tongue image, eye image and human breath have been imported from Traditional Chinese Medicine (TCM) and developed applicable diagnosis methods. To be mentioned in particular, diagnoses on diabetes based on human breath analysis have achieved higher accuracy on traditional ways such as urine test, without losing the advantage on high speed and low cost.

Finger-vein identification has been rising since around 2003, and soon become one of the top biometric identification techniques due to its significant performance on accuracy, speed, sanitation, maintenance and security. When it comes to medical purpose, finger-vein features are underneath but within shallow surface of human finger and are parts of human internal circulation system, which makes the features being able to directly reflecting physical conditions of human body, while at the same time remain easy to acquire. In this paper, we would discuss whether finger-vein features can be used as a valid indicator for human health conditions.

2   Defining Standard on Health Indicators

2.1   Analysis Popular Health Indicators

Nowadays, popular health indicators include heart rate, body temperature, PLT (blood platelet), RBC (red blood cell), WBC (white blood cell), BMI (body mass index), etc. After observations and comparisons among them, we here propose **Three Necessary Conditions** to become health indicators:

- CONDITION 1: **Relativity**. Indicators should have direct and accurate relativity to human health condition;
- CONDITION 2: **Stability in short term**. Indicators should be of dynamic balance in short term, which means although fluctuation of indicator does exist, it is within certain rage. After we decide a tested threshold based on enough data, indicators will achieve dynamic balance, or so called steady-state [2] with the given threshold;
- CONDITION 3: **Transformation in long term**. Indicators should correspond immediately when physiological condition of human body changes over long term, whether the change is positive or negative;

Based on these three necessary conditions, we can decide whether finger-vein features are able to make a valid health indicator. But first we have to make these three conditions more specific to our focused problem and quantified.

2.2 Three Necessary Conditions for Finger-Vein Features

To clear out, our finger-vein based system is a non-linear and non-continuous system. So there might not be perfect linear function for us to find out. And because studying a vector with high dimension like finger-vein image means unbearable large amount of work, so we project the images to low-dimensional space and focus on their distances between each other.

Under such premises, based on previous discussion, we now put the three necessary conditions a step forward:

Consider an autonomous nonlinear dynamical system [4] $\dot{X} = f(x(i)), x(0) = x_0$,

Where $x(i) \in D \subseteq \mathbb{R}^n$ denotes the mapped finger-vein image vector, D is an open set containing the mapped images, and $f:D \to \mathbb{R}^n$ non-continuous on D. Then we rewrite the three necessary conditions:

1. There is function as $\dot{X} = f(x(i))$, where $\dot{X}$ stands for human health condition, i stands for finger-vein images, and $x(i)$ stands for image after mapped to low-dimensional space. This function is non-continuous.

   Note that i is a finger-vein image and it should contain **PURE** information of finger-vein features, which means we should exclude exogenous variables such as influence of acquisition environment (illumination, temperature, humidity, etc.) or human factors (finger posture, dirty finger surface, etc.).

2. For this non-continuous function, we bring in variable of time t. Then for time t, there exists $\delta > 0$ such that

   If i_t, i_0 within time range δ, then $\left\| f\left(x\left(i_t\right)\right) - f\left(x\left(i_0\right)\right) \right\| < threshold$.

3. Average on $f(x(i))$ would change over long time span.

3   Evaluation Work on the Three Necessary Conditions

3.1 Preprocessing Data

Researchers use near-infrared light at 700–1000 nm wavelength to obtain finger-vein pictures. Acquiring devices are usually categorized into two types: reflection type and transmission type, as is shown in Fig. 1.

In this paper, we use 860 nm wavelength of near-infrared light and transmission type of acquisition device. As for algorithms, we choose wide line detector [5] to extract binary template from acquired finger-vein images.

After necessary adjustment (discussed hereinafter) has been made on cameras, finger-vein images are acquired in the format of 512 * 384 pixels, with each pixel being presented in 8 bits, as is shown in Fig. 2.

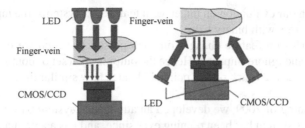

Fig. 1. Two types of acquisition devices

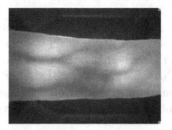

Fig. 2. Original finger-vein sample

As for the whole enroll process, we developed our algorithm in reference to Beining Huang's work in 2012 [6]. The processing steps are shown in Fig. 3:

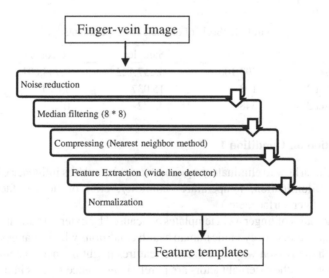

Fig. 3. Processing steps of finger-vein

After resizing the sample using nearest neighbor method, the format changes into 128 * 80 * 8 bits. At the end, the format of generated feature templates is binary image with size of 128 * 80.

Therefore, in our evaluation on finger-vein features in systems, the inputs of system are 128 * 80 vectors with binary value.

Since we focus on feature changes on each person itself, so we only concern on Genuine match and ignore Imposter. Hence the outputs are a set of points in a geometric space. Distance between each pair of points indicates how similar these two finger-vein samples are.

In the beginning of 2009, we developed an attendance system based on finger-vein verification. This system has been running ever since, and has accumulated so far more than 280,000 registered fingers, over 3,000,000 finger-vein samples, and 2,500,000 Genuine match recorded. We use this 7-years database as source of data as our **first** database.

We define "short term" as four years. If there are records of one finger during a specific time in the first dataset, we say this finger is active during that period. A rule has been made about finding fingers which are always active during autumn of 2013, spring of 2014, autumn of 2014 and spring of 2015. After traversing the first dataset, 108 fingers meet the rule, thus forming the **second** database.

As for Condition 3, we collect a group of samples from a group of more aged people:

1. 87 people in total;
2. 12 females, 65 males; Age range from 30 to 85;
3. 55 people are over 40.

We use same amount of young people (age range from 18 to 24) together to form the **third** dataset (Table 1).

Table 1. Scale of datasets for experiments

	Fingers	Samples	Records
Dataset 1	299,100	3,257,122	2,744,601
Dataset 2	108	15,037	14,701
Dataset 3	348	4,872	0

3.2   Evaluation on Condition 1

Critical work in on how to eliminate exogenous variables such as influence of acquisition environment (illumination, temperature, humidity, etc.) or human factors (finger posture, dirty finger surface, etc.).

Distance of pairs of finger-vein templates are caused by external and internal factors.

The internal factors are dynamic human health conditions which changes all the time. They are the direct reason why all biometric features might be inconsistent.

On the contrary, the external factors are purely interference factors in our study. We located three main external factors and corresponding work has been done to eliminate them:

1. Illumination fluctuation. When acquiring images, the illumination of environment affects the date mostly. Hence we add an illumination algorithm before the camera takes the image, which will adjust the grayscale distribution of the image by

controlling the near-infrared LED array. The adjusting algorithm builds on Shilei Liu's work in 2012 [7].

2. Posture change. The acquisition device is a 3-D device, thus making fingers unable to be located strictly. Shifting and rotation in any direction could cause significant difference on the geometric position of the newly acquired image, making finger-vein features appear to be inconsistent. We add a posture correction part during extraction, in reference to Beining Huang's work in 2012 [6].

3. Other environmental factors such as temperature, humidity, dust, etc. These factors are all potentially influential and very hard to study on the correlation. So we choose to study images which are acquired in a short period of time (usually within 30 s). In this way, influences from the environmental factors has been greatly impaired.

After eliminating these external factors, we are still able to observe fluctuation on finger-vein features, hence we can conclude finger-vein fulfils condition 1.

3.3   Evaluation on Condition 2

Dataset 2 is used to determine whether finger-vein features would change over short term (four years). The experiments results are as follows (Table 2):

Table 2.   Accumulated failure times for each finger

	Times	Percentage
Never	247,388	82.71%
At most 1 time	25,443	8.51%
At most 2 times	18,981	7.46%
More than 2	7,288	2.44%

Considering we are talking about accumulated times, the failure rate is quite low, hence proving finger-vein feature is stable in short term.

3.4   Evaluation on Condition 3

Since finger-vein study is young and currently we are not able to collect finger-vein images from the same person over more than 7 years. So we have to use a tricky way to conduct experiments of this part. We collect finger-vein images from young people and old people (dataset 3), and try to study if anything different between these two groups.

Referring to the idea of wide-line detector [5], we analyze the feature from vertical and horizontal directions (eight directions for each pixel). Experiments has shown two groups perform significantly different in finger-vein features. The young group have 63.22% features in horizontal directions, while the aged group only have 30.59%. Medical explanation is that when people are over 40, the vascular would begin to age, causing distortion occurs in vein.

4 Conclusion

In this paper, we propose three Necessary Conditions to become valid human health indicators. And conduct experiments on these three conditions to evaluate whether finger-vein features are capable of become on. The experiments have full shown that finger-vein features fulfil these three conditions, thus becoming a potential health indicator for human health. In the future, with more finger-vein image data attached with human physiological indexes, it is possible to build quantized mapping from vein image to specific parts of human health.

References

1. Jain, A., Bolle, R., Pankanti, S.: Biometrics: personal identification in networked society (2006)
2. Lyapunov, A.M.: The general problem of the stability of motion. Doctoral dissertation (1892)
3. Cattell, R.B.: Factor analysis: an introduction to essentials. The purpose and underlying models. Biometrics 21, 190–215 (1965)
4. Katok, A., Hasselblatt, B.: Introduction to the modern theory of dynamical systems (1995)
5. Liu, L., Zhang, D., You, J.: Detecting wide line using isotropic nonlinear filtering. IEEE Trans. Image Process. 15, 3608–3614 (2007)
6. Huang, B., Liu, S., Li, W.: A finger posture change correction method for finger-vein recognition. In: IEEE Symposium on Computational Intelligence for Security and Defense Applications (2012)
7. Liu, S., Huang, B., Yu, Y., Li, W.: Biometric identification system's performance enhancement by improving registration progress. In: The 7th Chinese Conference on Biometric Recognition (2012)

A Cluster Method to Noninvasive Continuous Blood Pressure Measurement Using PPG

Yu Miao, Zhiqiang Zhang[✉], Lifang Meng, Xiaoqin Xie, and Haiwei Pan

College of Computer Science and Technology, Harbin Engineering University,
Nantong Street no.145, Harbin 150001, China
zqzhang@hrbeu.edu.cn

Abstract. Blood pressure (BP) is an important physiological signal of human body. How to measure blood pressure is a meaningful problem for detection of human health. The most commonly used method is cuff based method. But this method can not used for continuous blood pressure measurement. For this concern, a Photoplethysmogram-based method for continuous blood pressure measurement was presented. Many researches have found that there are some relations exist between some Photoplethysmogram (PPG) signal features and human blood pressure. We use an artificial neural network model and a cluster method to make some estimation on human blood pressure based on Photoplethysmogram signal, and our result shows that this method can be used for noninvasive continuous blood pressure measurement in future.

Keywords: Blood pressure · Photoplethysmogram · Artificial neural network · Cluster

1 Introduction

Blood pressure is an important physiological signal of human body. Normal blood pressure is a prerequisite for the circulation of the blood flow, blood pressure remained normal under the regulation in a variety of factors, so as to provide various organs with sufficient blood and maintain the normal process of metabolism. Blood pressure measurement is an important tool for assessment of the clinical condition of patients and is necessary to predict the future cardiovascular and overall health. However, the measurement ways only provide a single average measurement; the measured value does not accurately reflect the true blood pressure level and cardiovascular status of the patients [1]. Continuous blood pressure measurement can monitor the changes of blood pressure in real time, and can help to evaluate the effect of antihypertensive drugs on patients. Automated non-invasive BP monitoring using Oscillometry [2] has become increasingly popular in recent years as it can relatively easily implemented in automated BP measurement device. Oscillometry is performed by inflating a cuff to a pressure above the systolic (SP) and then deflating it to a pressure below the diastolic blood pressure (DP). However, long time inflating and deflating will make person uncomfortable. It's necessary to have a measurement way of non-invasive and continual to estimate blood pressure.

© Springer International Publishing AG 2017
C. Xing et al. (Eds.): ICSH 2016, LNCS 10219, pp. 109–120, 2017.
DOI: 10.1007/978-3-319-59858-1_11

This paper contains 5 parts: We make a brief introduction for blood pressure measurement in part 1, and then describe some related work about noninvasive blood pressure estimation next part. In part 3, we introduce our pretreatment and feature extraction method. In part 4, we present how our estimation model builds. An experimental result is given in part 5. In final part, we make a conclusion for our work. Our workflow can be seen in Fig. 1.

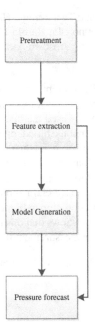

Fig. 1. Blood estimation work flow

2   Related Work

Nowadays, the most common way to measure blood pressure is based on cuff [3]. This method estimate the blood pressure based on Korotkoff sound judgment [4]. There is no sound when blood flows in the blood vessels, but when the blood passes through the narrow blood vessels to form a vortex, the sound can be made. In the measurement, we should fix the cuff to the brachial artery, and exert pressure to the cuff, and then we can adjust the pressure in the cuff to monitor the Korotkoff sound, so as to achieve the purpose of measuring blood pressure.

The blood measurement method based on cuff can not used for continuous measurement because its inconvenience and the cuff may cause the discomfort of the person being tested. Later, due to the development of light spot sensor, some new measurement methods have been proposed. Some researches have found that Pulse Wave Velocity (PWV) has a close relationship with blood pressure, so 'The Pulse Wave Velocity measurement [5–8]' has been presented. For the realization of the PWV based blood pressure trend tracking, the Pulse Transit Time (PTT) is needed. Many people have mentioned the method based photoelectric Photoplethysmogram and Electrocardiograph (ECG). FS Cattivelli and H Garudadri use a Pulse Arrival Time (PAT) to replace PTT [9]. Besides, others use two PPG sensor replace ECG for blood pressure measurement [10]. Indeed, if you get a high quality ECG and fingertip pulse waveform, there is a good chance that you can get a good result. However, the photoelectric PPG wearable devices have a weak anti-interference ability, and there is a big problem in the quality of the photoelectric signal and the signal quality will directly affect the calculation accuracy of follow-up.

Except PWV, 'pulse wave characteristic parameter determination method [11–15]' has also been presented. While the second method of measurement BP only request a PPG signal and it is convenient for real-time measurement. The human body's pulse wave can reflect the physiological state of the human body as a whole, so the abundant information contained in the pulse wave is of great medical value. This blood pressure measurement method is that making use of the characteristics of the pulse wave to calculate the body's blood pressure. Some representative features have been found from the PPG signal, and many researchers think these features have close relations with blood pressure. The general steps: extraction of human pulse wave; and then extract the characteristics of pulse wave and the analysis of the related human blood pressure level; finally, select features which have high correlation with blood pressure and estimate blood pressure. At present, many researchers have studied this kind of measurement method, which can realize continuous single cycle measurement. Therefore, this kind of measurement method has great potential and good prospect. To sum up, many researchers have made some achievements in noninvasive measurement of blood pressure. There is still much room for development.

Therefore, this article will study the nonivasive blood pressure measurement based on photoelectric pulse wave, using 4 pulse wave characteristic parameters obtained from PPG which have the highest correlation with blood pressure. Then, In order to obtain the complex relationships between these features and blood pressure, we build an artificial neural network (ANN) model to realize it. We use a cluster method to optimize blood pressure estimation process, and put forward effective solutions to the problems in the realization process.

3   Pretreatment and Feature Extraction

3.1   Pretreatment

The Photoplethysmogram signal contains many meaningful features; researchers have found that the quality of the PPG signal is influenced by many factors, including the individual skin structure, the blood oxygen saturation, blood flow rate, skin temperatures and the measuring environment [16].

In most cases, the original signal contains various noises caused by these factors. So, for getting accurate features, many filter methods have been proposed. Most papers use a wavelet to filter the original signal for its good performance. But for our signal data, we found that different sample has different noise, and their noise rates and shapes varies

sharply. In order to get a general usable filter result, we use a moving average method
to filter the original signal.

3.2 Feature Extraction

A large number of features have been found by others, but they extract features for
Specific signals with specific shapes. Millasseau S C, et al. classify PPG signals into 4
classes (e.g. contains dicrotic wave or not, dicrotic wave is clear or not) in [17], the
signal changes with age, gender and other human body factors. Different types are
included in our data set (Fig. 2), so most specific features extraction methods can not be
used. However, no matter what type the signal is, they must have a main wave that
represents the main pulse change. As a result, we extract 4 essential features, which can
be seen in Fig. 3.

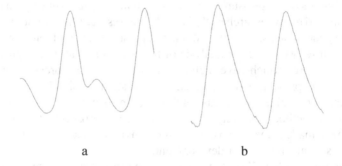

a   b

Fig. 2. PPG signals of different class

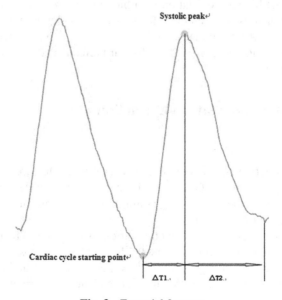

Fig. 3. Essential features

- **Cardiac cycle starting point:** we extract the cardiac cycle starting point as the first feature, it is the first point and the lowest amplitude point of a cardiac cycle, it reflects the lowest pulse pressure.
- **Systolic peak:** systolic peak is the highest amplitude point of a cardiac cycle, and it is the maximum pressure point of pulse pressure.
- **Systolic period:** expressed as $\triangle T1$ reflect the contraction time of blood vessel.
- **Diastolic period:** expressed as $\triangle T2$ reflect the diastolic time of blood vessel.

These 4 features can be seen as 2 points, so we need to find these 2 points at each cardiac cycle. In order to get these 2 points, we have a process to deal with the signal.

Firstly, we need to calculate the cycle of the signal. Most used methods to get cycle of a signal are fast Fourier transform and wavelet transform. In this paper we use fast Fourier transform to get cycle, it can transform time domain signal to frequency domain, and the maximum amplitude of frequency domain signal correspond to the main frequency component. And we can get cycle though the main frequency (i.e. the reciprocal of the main frequency).

Secondly, we will find all the maximum value and the minimum value. This process can be done by calculating the PPG signal's first-order derivative. It is worth noting that, because the signal is discrete, we can not simply seek the zero points of first-order derivative. Therefore, we first calculate first-order difference of original signal, and then use a sign function to deal with them, and we get all 1 represent rising stage of signal and -1 represent falling stage of signal. Now, we can calculate difference again and all -2 values represent maximum values and all 2 values represent minimum values.

Then, we need judge whether a signal have dicrotic wave. This can be realized by comparing the general cycle and the mean of any 2 successive maximum values or minimum values. After that, we can divide the whole signal into numerous cardiac cycles, and the first minimum value and first maximum value correspond to the 2 main points.

Finally, through some statistical methods we can remove the abnormal feature points consist of abnormal amplitude and abnormal time period.

4   Model Generation

4.1   Experimental Data Set

Before the model generation, we gave an outline of our data set. We get data from mimic.physionet.org. The MIMIC database is composed of two distinctive groups of data. The clinical database and high resolution waveforms recorded database [18]. MIMIC is a valuable resource, especially for those researchers who do not have easy access to the clinical intensive care environment [19]. In the data set, we have over 4000 sets of data, each set contains PPG signal whose whole time period is 600 s and sampling frequency is 100 Hz, and standard SP and DP values obtained from standard medical equipment which sampling frequency is not certain. Each set represent a different patient and we can use the PPG signal to build model and use the SP and DP value as the standard output data.

4.2 Artificial Neural Network Model

Previous related work has shown that some linear correlations between blood pressure and some features [20]. But based on our data set these linear correlations shows poor effect, and can not be used to estimate blood pressure. So we think between the PPG signal and blood pressure there is a more complex correlation which can not be simply discovered. For this purpose, we use an artificial neural network to build a model.

We build a network with 2 hidden layers and 4 inputs and 2 outputs. Different evaluation indicators often have different dimension and dimension units, so that the situation will affect the results of the data analysis. So before training the network model, we have carried on the normalization processing to the data, in order to eliminate the influence of dimension between indexes. And we use a Min-Max Normalization method to do such thing; its formula can be seen in Eq. (1). X indicates an arbitrary feature vector, and Xmin indicates the minimum value in X, Xmax indicates the maximum value in X. through this method we can normalize features to 0–1 range and speed up the convergence of the model.

$$X^* = (X - Xmin)/(Xmax - Xmin) \tag{1}$$

In general, it is understandable that different person has different factors except pulse signal and these factors can also influence their blood pressure. So we have reasons to believe that different person have different correlation between blood pressure and PPG signal features. So we should build different model for different person. But on the other hand, in reality, for many reasons, we can not get enough data of every person while the greater the amount of data, the artificial neural network obtains more accurate results. We think build a unified model for all people may be feasible. We tried these 2 ways on our data set. The result can be seen in Table 1.

Table 1. Individual model result

SP standard deviation	Ratio	DP standard deviation	Ratio
e < 5	0.709	e < 5	0.918
e < 8	0.864	e < 8	0.965
e < 10	0.906	e < 10	0.977

For the individual model, we chose sequential 80% data of every individual person's signal for training network, and the remaining data for testing our model performance. For every 4 features in every cycle, our model will give 2 outputs correspond to systolic pressure and diastolic pressure. Comparing to the standard blood pressure values, we can get the errors of each estimation. Then the standard deviation of each individual test set was calculated using all the errors. For the unified model, we chose sequential 80% data of every individual person's signal and combine them together for training a unified network, and similarly, we got the standard deviation of each individual test set (Table 2).

Table 2. Unified model result

SP standard deviation	Ratio	DP standard deviation	Ratio
e < 5	0.139	e < 5	0.290
e < 8	0.263	e < 8	0.469
e < 10	0.335	e < 10	0.580

From the table, we confirm that the unified model had a worse result compare to the individual model. Besides, we found the standard deviation of DP is lower than SP, it may suggest that these features are more closely related to diastolic blood pressure. In order to solving the contradiction between data quantity and accuracy, we propose a cluster method to solve this problem.

4.3 Model Combined with Cluster Method

To make a trade-off between data quantity and accuracy, we combine all individual people's signal together and then use a cluster algorithm to divide them into different cluster. Next, for every cluster we make a neural network model, and use this model to estimate new arrival signal data that belongs to the same cluster.

For the cluster method we adjust the features numbers from 4 to 3, in other words, we use an amplitude difference to replace starting point amplitude and systolic peak amplitude because these 2 amplitudes vary with multiple external factors. So we use the relative value instead of the absolute value to process the cluster. Our experimental result can be seen in next part.

5 Experimental Result

In order to test the effect of the model, we made an experiment for our cluster estimation model. In the experiment, we chose 100 groups of PPG signal, put them together and run a cluster algorithm on 80% of them and get corresponding network model of each cluster. Then we can get the performance of this method. We set the number of clusters, K, from 5 to 10, and use two frequently-used methods which are k-means and k-medoids to execute our experiment. 4 distance functions are used in our cluster method, they are Euler distance, Manhattan distance, cosine distance and correlation distance. Because the cluster algorithm and the neural network have some uncertainty, we make 3 tests for every different parameter.

Our result is shown in Figs. 4, 5, 6 and 7. The unified standard deviation of 100 groups has been got, and standard deviation of SP and DP respectively is 12.286 and 6.967. From our result we can see that all the standard deviation obtained from our cluster method are lower than the unified standard deviation and with the change of K value, there is no uniform law exist. For 4 distance functions, Euler distance and Manhattan distance are much better than cosine distance and correlation distance. Besides, k-medoids has much better performance than K-means.

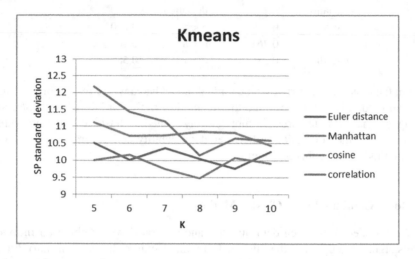

Fig. 4. SP standard deviation among different K value on K-means method

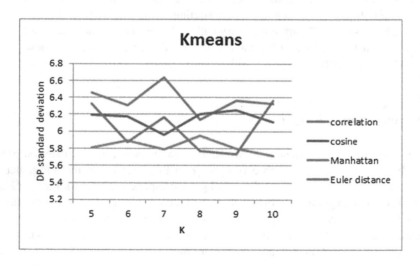

Fig. 5. DP standard deviation among different K value on K-means method

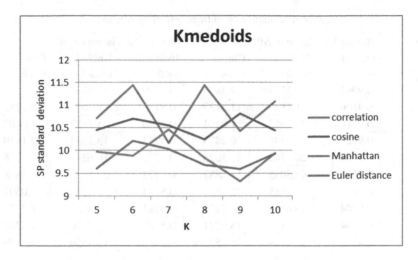

Fig. 6. SP standard deviation among different K value on K-medoids method

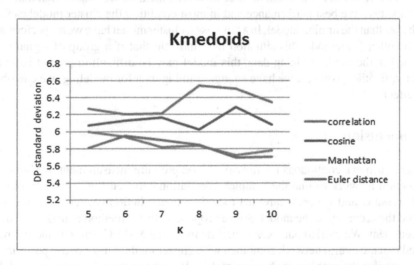

Fig. 7. DP standard deviation among different K value on K-medoids method

Next we compare the cluster method model with the individual model. We use k-medoids algorithm and set distance function as Euler distance and K fixed to 8. Then chose 10 additional groups signal data, and use the cluster estimation models to estimate these data of 10 groups. We can compare this result with the result obtained from individual model. The result is shown in Table 3.

Table 3. Comparison of three modeling method

Order	Standard deviation of SP			Standard deviation of DP		
	Individual model	Unified model	Cluster model	Individual model	Unified model	Cluster model
1	0.9091	8.3124	4.3876	0.5710	18.5638	3.7414
2	0.9106	21.4849	11.5137	0.5715	8.7652	5.5285
3	0.9116	12.9962	1.0464	0.5750	15.7127	1.0402
4	0.9129	23.5198	20.2475	0.5753	13.3383	12.1819
5	0.9148	26.3742	42.5025	0.5772	16.6241	23.9028
6	0.9160	44.3055	11.8887	0.5772	27.1037	6.7878
7	0.9184	2.7985	42.1861	0.5784	2.0534	34.0507
8	0.9204	26.4191	6.7424	0.5784	17.8611	28.4731
9	0.9204	16.2899	18.9221	0.5787	4.7170	9.4778
10	0.9208	16.4648	1.7573	0.5796	12.4556	1.5899

From the result in comparison of three modeling method, we can see that individual model always have best performance and in most condition the cluster model can estimate better than the unified model. In a few cases, cluster model have worse performance than the other 2 method. This situation may indicate that if a group of signal is not contained in the model training data, this model may be difficult to predict its output correctly, in other words, if we have enough training data for modeling, we can obtain good effect.

6   Conclusion

In order to achieve continuous noninvasive blood pressure measurement, we build artificial neural network to find the complex correlation between PPG signal and human blood pressure, and we are aware that there is a contradiction between the amount of data and the accuracy of the model. So we propose a cluster method to make a trade-off between them. We carried out some experiments on the MIMIC data set, and our result showed that the neural network combined with cluster method has a better performance and it can solve the problem of shortage of data. Because of the privacy of medical data, it is difficult for us to get enough experimental data and we can not obtain some other personal information about person. In other words, if there is some other detailed information, we can treat them as additional features and combine them together to train models, and we have reasons to believe that it can get much better results.

Acknowledgments. This work is supported by the National Natural Science Foundation of China (Nos. 61672181, 61202090, 61272184), Natural Science Foundation of Heilongjiang Province (No. F2016005), the Science and Technology Innovation Talents Special Fund of Harbin (Nos. 2016RAXXJ036, 2015RQQXJ067), the opening found of Key Laboratory of Machine Perception (Ministry of Education), Peking University (K-2016-02).

References

1. Fortino, G., Giampà, V.: PPG-based methods for non invasive and continuous blood pressure measurement: an overview and development issues in body sensor networks. In: IEEE International Workshop on Medical Measurements and Applications Proceedings, pp. 10–13 (2010)
2. Barbe, K., Van Moer, W., Schoors, D.: Analyzing the windkessel model as a potential candidate for correcting oscillometric blood-pressure measurements. IEEE Trans. Instrum. Meas. **61**(2), 411–418 (2012)
3. Rd, R.M.: Noninvasive automatic determination of mean arterial pressure. Med. Biol. Eng. Comput. **17**(1), 11–18 (1979)
4. Drzewiecki, G.M., Melbin, J., Noordergraaf, A.: The Korotkoff sound. Ann. Biomed. Eng. **17**(4), 325–359 (1989)
5. Muehlsteff, J., Aubert, X.L., Schuett, M.: Cuffless estimation of systolic blood pressure for short effort bicycle tests: the prominent role of the pre-ejection period. In: Conference Proceedings: Annual International Conference of the IEEE Engineering in Medicine and Biology Society, pp. 5088–5092 (2006)
6. Kachuee, M., Kiani, M.M., Mohammadzade, H., et al.: Cuff-less high-accuracy calibration-free blood pressure estimation using pulse transit time. In: IEEE International Symposium on Circuits and Systems, pp. 1006–1009. IEEE (2015)
7. Gu, W.B., Poon, C.C.Y., Zhang, Y.T.: A novel parameter from PPG dicrotic notch for estimation of systolic blood pressure using pulse transit time. In: International Summer School and Symposium on Medical Devices and Biosensors, Isss-Mdbs, pp. 86–88. IEEE (2008)
8. Meigas, K., Kattai, R., Lass, J.: Continuous blood pressure monitoring using pulse wave delay. In: Proceedings of the International Conference of the IEEE Engineering in Medicine and Biology Society, vol. 4, pp. 3171–3174 (2001)
9. Cattivelli, F.S., Garudadri, H.: Noninvasive cuffless estimation of blood pressure from pulse arrival time and heart rate with adaptive calibration. In: International Workshop on Wearable and Implantable Body Sensor Networks, BSN 2009, Berkeley, CA, USA, 3–5 June, pp. 114–119 (2009)
10. Bhavirisetty, R.T.: Calculation of blood pulse transit time from PPG (2012)
11. Hassan, M.K.B.A., Mashor, M.Y., Nasir, N.F.M., et al.: Measuring blood pressure using a photoplethysmography approach. Ifmbe Proc. **21**(1), 591–594 (2007)
12. Yan, Y.S., Zhang, Y.T.: Noninvasive estimation of blood pressure using photoplethysmographic signals in the period domain. In: Conference Proceedings of the Annual International Conference of the IEEE Engineering in Medicine and Biology Society, pp. 3583–3584. IEEE Engineering in Medicine and Biology Society (2005)
13. Kurylyak, Y., Lamonaca, F., Grimaldi, D.: A neural network-based method for continuous blood pressure estimation from a PPG signal. In: Conference Record - IEEE Instrumentation and Measurement Technology Conference, vol. 80(11), pp. 280–283 (2013)
14. Gunasekaran, V.: Continuous non-invasive arterial blood pressure measurement using photoplethysmography. Electronic Theses & Dissertations (2013)
15. Yoon, Y.Z., Yoon, G.W.: Nonconstrained blood pressure measurement by photoplethysmography. J. Opt. Soc. Korea **10**(2), 91–95 (2006)
16. Elgendi, M.: On the analysis of fingertip Photoplethysmogram signals. Curr. Cardiol. Rev. **8**(1), 14–25 (2012)
17. Millasseau, S.C., Ritter, J.M., Takazawa, K., et al.: Contour analysis of the photoplethysmographic pulse measured at the finger. J. Hypertens. **24**(8), 1449–1456 (2006)

18. Clifford, G.D., Scott, D.J., Villarroel, M., et al.: User guide and documentation for the MIMIC II database. Mimic (2009)
19. Lee, J., Scott, D.J., Villarroel, M., et al.: Open-access MIMIC-II database for intensive care research. In: International Conference of the IEEE Engineering in Medicine & Biology Society, pp. 8315–8318 (2011)
20. Samria, R., Jain, R., Jha, A., et al.: Noninvasive cuff'less estimation of blood pressure using Photoplethysmography without electrocardiograph measurement. In: Region 10 Symposium, pp. 254–257. IEEE (2014)

A Multi-feature Fusion Method to Estimate Blood Pressure by PPG

Lifang Meng, Zhiqiang Zhang$^{(\boxtimes)}$, Yu Miao, Xiaoqin Xie, and Haiwei Pan

College of Computer Science and Technology, Harbin Engineering University,
Nantong Street No. 145, Harbin 150001, China
zqzhang@hrbeu.edu.cn

Abstract. Effective features extracted from Photoplethysmogram (PPG) are the central for estimating accurately blood pressure (BP). To make extracted features have a strong correlation with real blood pressure, a model based on feature fusion is presented to evaluate blood pressure. To divide pulse wave into two types of dicrotic wave and non-dicrotic wave, different types of waveforms use different extracted features, and wavelet transform is used to remove the noise from the extracted features. Linear regression model and neural network are evaluation models, and Matlab system identification toolboxes are used to recognize the model parameters. The experiment results have shown that extracted features have a correlation with systolic pressure (SP) and diastolic pressure (DP). The value of blood pressure can be calculated based on features extracted from PPG. What's more, the accuracy of the fusion feature model is improved compared with the traditional method only by using one type of extracted feature method for all the pulse waveforms.

Keywords: Blood pressure · Photoplethysmogram · Dicrotic wave · Linear regression · Neural network

1 Introduction

Blood pressure is the side pressure of blood on the unit area blood vessels when blood flows in the blood vessels. In addition, it is an important physiological parameter to reflect the function of the human body circulatory system [1], and to predict the future cardiovascular and overall health. Monitoring blood pressure in real-time and analyzing the obtained data can evaluate a person's cardiovascular function in a period, and make reasonable and correct diagnosis and treatment in time, which can prevent the occurrence of cardiovascular disease in a way. Nowadays, the blood pressure measurement device that is used in hospital and family is mainly oscillometric-based method [2]. Oscillometry can accurately measure blood pressure with cuff, and oscillometry performed by inflating a cuff to a pressure above the systolic (SP) and then deflating it to a pressure below the diastolic blood pressure (DP), and it is not a method for continuous monitoring of blood pressure. In addition, the cuff will make the subjects to measure on the arm or wrist position measuring pressure, and make the subjects feel uncomfortable [3]. It is necessary to have a non-invasive [4] and continual measurement way to estimate blood pressure.

C. Xing et al. (Eds.): ICSH 2016, LNCS 10219, pp. 121–131, 2017.
DOI: 10.1007/978-3-319-59858-1_12

This paper contains 5-parts: A brief introduction for blood pressure measurement will be presented in part one, and then describes some related work about non-invasive blood pressure estimation next part. The third part will show selected features and feature extraction methods. In part four, we will demonstrate our choice of the evaluation model and explain how to conduct the experiment, and the experimental result is given in this part. In final part, we make a conclusion for our work and our future work.

2   Related Work

At present, the mainly methods focus on the use of ECG and PPG two kinds of periodic signal [5, 6]. In recent decades, many research efforts have been expended in the field of non-invasive, continuous BP estimation by cardiovascular surrogate parameters, mainly the pulse transit time (PTT) and pulse transit velocity [7–14]. However, the BP predictions PTT-based requires PPG with an additional measurement of electrocardiogram (ECG) which requires the attachment of electrodes on the surface of human body. Indeed, if you get a high quality ECG and photoelectric signal PPG reflecting pulse waveform, there is a good chance that you can get a good result. However, in order to accomplish a completely non-constrained measurement, we investigated a method of predicting BP without ECG from only one periodic signal PPG waveform.

PPG is a non-invasive electro-optical signal, which gives information about the volume of blood flowing through the body testing zone, close to the skin. It is convenient for real-time measurement. The human body's pulse wave can reflect the physiological state of the human body as a whole, so the abundant information contained in the pulse wave is of great medical value [15]. Showed that there was a complex relation, not always linear, between the blood pressure and pulse wave obtained from PPG signal. And it use the Artificial Neural Networks(ANNs) model to estimate BP, and extracted 21 parameters in each cycle from every periodic signal PPG waveform as the input vector for the ANN. However, this feature extraction method of 21 parameters is only suitable for the waveform without the dicrotic wave, and the waveform with dicrotic wave by 21 parameters will show very poor effect. [16, 17] these papers devoted themselves to committing to the pulse wave transform from the time domain into frequency domain, and extracted features from the spectrum. [18, 19] these papers studied some features extracted from only PPG, which can reflect well on physiological significance. These blood pressure measurement methods are that making use of the features of the pulse wave to calculate the body's blood pressure. The general steps: obtain human pulse wave, and then extract the characteristics of pulse wave and the analysis of the related human blood pressure level; finally, select features that have a strong correlation with real blood pressure. Many researchers have identified PPG have different waveforms in different time or different situation, but there are fewer researches on which different waveforms made use of different extracted features, which can realize continuous single cycle more accurately measurement so far. Therefore, a fusion-based measurement has great potential and good prospect. To sum up, many researchers have made some achievements in noninvasive measurement of blood pressure. There is still much room for development.

Therefore, this paper will study the non-invasive blood pressure measurement based on PPG, using pulse wave feature parameters obtained from PPG, which have the highest correlation with blood pressure, and put forward effective solutions to the problems in the realization process.

3   Feature Parameters

In this paper, the block diagram for BP estimation was shown in Fig. 1, which consists of the following steps: (1) experiment data source block to select a database with adequate sample size. (2) Preprocessing block to smooth and remove invalid signal. (3) Classify PPG signal block to divide all PPG waveforms into two types of waveforms, dicrotic wave and without dicrotic wave. (4) Determining methods of extraction feature block to extract useful features from different type signals. (5) Partitioning block to partition the samples in three subsets i.e. train, validation and test. (6) Machine Learning block to train the regression models. (7) Evaluation model block to evaluate the trained models' performance. (8) The cooperation of 21-feature parameters and 13-feature parameters block to show the experiment results. All these steps are discussed in detail in the sequel.

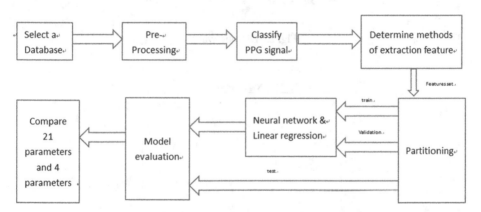

Fig. 1. Estimation BP processing block diagram

3.1   Pre-processing

The first block of database will give a detailed description in the experimental section. PPG signal uses the photoelectric sensor to detect the difference of the reflected light intensity after the body's blood and tissue absorption. In addition, it traces out the blood vessel volume in the cardiac cycle changes from the pulse waveform to calculate the BP. PPG signal obtained from photoelectric sensor contains some noise, we use wavelet transform for filtering and removing baseline drift. With the increment of the decomposition, the high frequency part the gradually reduce, and the low frequency part gradually increase. Therefore, we use wavelet basic function db5 to filter noise.

3.2 Classify PPG Signal and Extract Features

PPG signal have different waveforms not only between different people, but also in different time, so it is very important to take different feature extraction methods for different waveforms to accurately estimate BP. According to the physiological significance of the pulse wave, the dicrotic wave is used as the criterion of the division. Figure 2 shows dicrotic wave, and Fig. 3 gives non-dicrotic wave.

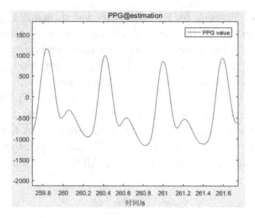

Fig. 2. Dicrotic wave

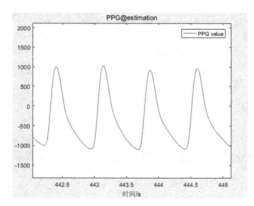

Fig. 3. Non-dicrotic wave

We first obtain PPG from database, extract all the peaks in the PPG signal, obtain the time interval values between the peaks, and finally, get the threshold by adaptive threshold method. PPG waveform can be divided different waveforms according to statistical threshold time interval. The next content will clearly illustrate the extracted features.

21-Feature Parameters

Although [15] have mentioned dicrotic waveform, the 21-feature cannot deal with this situation. The features are given as Fig. 4.

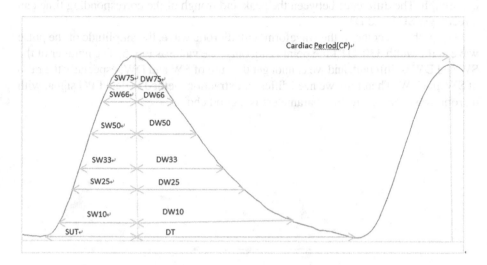

Fig. 4. 21-feature parameters

Many researches have studied that the amplitude of pulse wave has less correlation with BP. In order to cover the whole pulse wave information well, the 21-feature are as follows:

Systolic upstroke time (SUT): Cardiac systolic part. (The time interval of amplitude from minimal to the maximal point)

Diastolic time (DT): Cardiac diastolic part. (The time interval of amplitude from maximal to next minimal point)

SW10, SW25, SW33, SW50, SW66, and SW75: get the time point that the width at 25%, 33%, 50%, 66%, 75% of SUT, and get the amplitude of the pulse wave at this time point.

DW10, DW25, DW33, DW50, DW66, and DW75: get the time point that the width at 25%, 33%, 50%, 66%, 75% of DT, and get the amplitude of the pulse wave at this time point.

CP: a single period of heartbeat.

21-features parameters also contains the times of systolic, diastolic parts and ratio between them. They are listed as follows:

CP, SUT, DT
At 10%: SW10, DW10, SW10 + DW10, DW10/SW10
At 25%: SW25, DW25, SW25 + DW25, DW25/SW25
At 33%: SW33, DW33, SW33 + DW33, DW33/SW33
At 50%: SW50, DW50, SW50 + DW50, DW50/SW50
At 66%: SW66, DW66, SW66 + DW66, DW66/SW66
At 75%: SW75, DW75, SW75 + DW75, DW75/SW75

The 21-feature parameters are obtained by the method. Get all peaks and troughs of the PPG signal, and store them in different matrix. Adaptive threshold method can help us easily get the every heartbeat period time (CT). In each period, there is only one peak and trough. The difference between the peak and trough of the corresponding time can directly get SUT and DT.

The problems come. If the waveform with dicrotic wave, the amplitude of the pulse wave at the width 33% DT time point is not only one value as Fig. 5. The number of the SW and DW is different, and we cannot get the sum of SW and DW, especially the ratio of SW and DW. Therefore, we need different extraction method to deal PPG signal with dicrotic wave, and 13-feature parameters is a good choice.

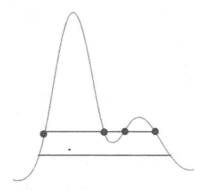

Fig. 5. Dicrotic wave correspond to many values

13-Feature Parameters

To solve above-mentioned challenges, we want to use some simple and significant features to treat with PPG signal with dicrotic wave. Therefore, we chose 13-feature parameters. Figure 6 picks up the significant features from the PPG.

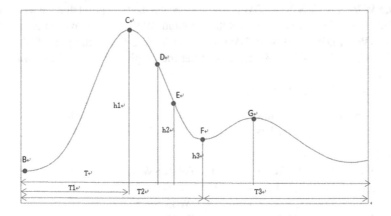

Fig. 6. 13-feature parameters

There are many researches on those feature parameters [20–23]. D, E, F, G feature points make full use of the physiological significance of the PPG signal generation. All of the 13-feature parameters are follows:

B: PPG signal trough. (Marks the beginning of the cardiac ejection period)
C: systolic peak
D: tidal wave (The left ventricular ejection shocks the artery to cause elastic vibration)
E: the boundary of systolic and diastolic
F: dicrotic notch
G: dicrotic peak
h1, h2/h1, h3/h1: relative height of amplitude
T: a complete waveform period
T1/T: systolic time ratio
T2/T: diastolic time ratio
H(1 + T1/T2): a physical signal of cardiac output 13-feature parameters can solve 21-feature parameters' problems well.

4 Evaluation Models and Experiment

4.1 Experiment Data

Before introducing our evaluation model, the part will give the experimental data source in brief. MIMIC is an openly available dataset developed by the MIT Lab for computational physiology, comprising identified health data associated with >40000 critical care patients. It includes demographics, vital signs, laboratory tests, medications, and more. You can get the data here: https://physionet.org/works/MIMICIIIClinicalDatabase/access.shtml. The next part will give the detail experiment results by linear regression and neural network.

4.2 Neural Network

There is not a very clear correlation about blood pressure and extracted features. ANN dealing with complex relations always performs well. The neural network is established with two hidden layers and two outputs (SP and DP). Note that the input of ANN is different. If the PPG signal have dicrotic wave, ANN needs 13 inputs, and PPG signal without dicrotic wave just provide 21 parameters to ANN as input. Different person have different correlation between blood pressure and PPG signal features. [15] Had product an experiment to get a reasonable result that the optimal architecture is {35, 20} with two hidden layers–35 neurons on the first hidden layer and 20 on the second one. Our experiment contains three parts: only use 21-feature parameters (just pick the first amplitude value to avoid above problem); only use 13-feature parameters (pick four of 13-feature parameters to deal with PPG signal with dicrotic wave); combine 13-feature parameters for PPG with dicrotic wave and 21-feature parameters for PPG without dicrotic wave. Compare estimated SP and real DP in the Fig. 7. Figure 8 shows estimated DP and real DP. Moreover, the errors are in Table 1.

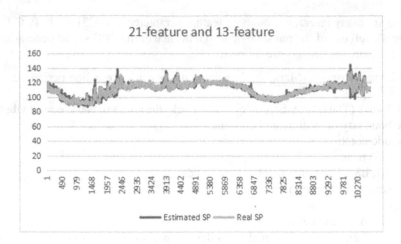

Fig. 7. Estimated SP and real SP

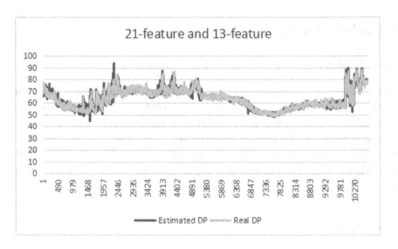

Fig. 8. Estimated DP and real DP

Table 1. The standard deviation of three methods

Methods	SP std	DP std
13-feature parameters	3.01	1.89
21-feature parameters	2.77	2.51
13-feature and 21-feature parameters	2.32	1.87

The experiment results have shown that neural network predict blood pressure well, the estimated BP fit real BP well. The standard deviations of all of the method are within 3, but the classification of pulse wave plays an important role in the physiological study of clinical medicine. However, the model still needs to improve the

learning ability of the blood pressure changing sharply, which is also very important in the practical application.

4.3   Linear Regression

There are so many researches on linear regression, some results showed the effect well,
and some of the results performed poorly. Therefore, linear regression is used to compare
with neural network according to 13-feature parameters and 21-feature parameters.
Compare estimated SP and real SP in the Fig. 9. Figure 10 gives estimated DP and real
DP. Moreover, the errors are in Table 2.

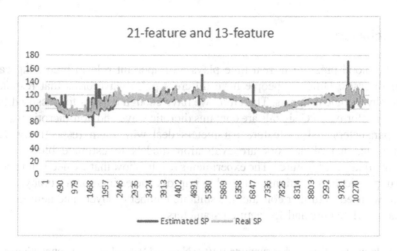

Fig. 9. Estimated SP and real SP

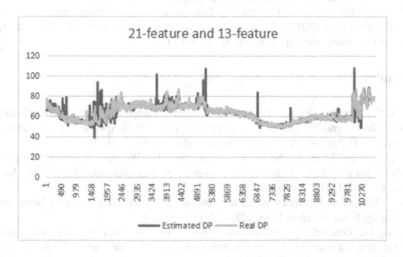

Fig. 10. Estimated DP and real DP

Table 2. The standard deviation of three methods

Methods	SP std	DP std
13-feature parameters	3.03	2.87
21-feature parameters	3.24	2.75
13-feature and 21-feature parameters	2.48	2.16

The experiment results reveal that neural network is more appropriate model. Despite that, all of the standard deviations are around 3, but the estimated blood pressure is very unstable. Some estimated values are far from real values. This is a great hidden danger in the practical application.

5   Conclusion

Estimating blood pressure in real time plays an important role in predicting cardiovascular diseases. Different people have different pulse waveforms that response to different physiological signals. Therefore, we have enough reasons to classify different types of waveforms. PPG signals are contains dicrotic wave and non-dicrotic wave. 21-feature parameters and 13-feature parameters deal with them respectively. Linear regression and neural network are evaluation models to estimate blood pressure according to extracted features. The experiments results show that we need more consideration in practical applications and need to improve the estimation accuracy.

Next, we need to further consider the suitable number of layers and neurons for the combination 21-feature and 13-feature parameters.

Acknowledgments. This work is supported by the National Natural Science Foundation of China (No. 61672181, 61202090, 61272184), Natural Science Foundation of Heilongjiang Province (No. F2016005), the Science and Technology Innovation Talents Special Fund of Harbin (No. 2016RAXXJ 036, 2015RQQXJ067), the opening found of Key Laboratory of Machine Perception (Ministry of Education), Peking University (K-2016-02).

References

1. Gu, Y.Y, Zhang, Y., Zhang, Y.T.: A novel biometric approach in human verification by photoplethysmographic signals. In: International IEEE EMBS Special Topic Conference on Information Technology Applications in Biomedicine, pp. 13–14 (2003)
2. Barbe, K., Van, Moer W., Schoors, D.: Analyzing the Windkessel model as a potential candidate for correcting oscillometric blood-pressure measurements. IEEE Trans. Instrum. Meas. **61**(2), 411–418 (2012)
3. Kim, J., Kim, W.S.: A paired stretchable printed sensor system for ambulatory blood pressure monitoring. Sens. Actuators Phys. **238**, 329–336 (2016)
4. Fortino, G., Giampà, V.: PPG-based methods for non invasive and continuous BP measurement: an overview and development issues in body sensor networks. In: Proceedings of IEEE International Workshop on Medical Measurements and Applications (MeMeA 2010), Ottawa, pp. 10–13 (2010)

5. Biel, L., Pettersson, O., Philipson, L., et al.: ECG analysis: a new approach in human identification. IEEE Trans. Instrum. Meas. **50**(3), 808–812 (2001)
6. Hegde, C., Prabhu, H.R., Sagar, D.S., et al.: Statistical analysis for human authentication using ECG waves. Commun. Comput. Inf. Sci. **141**, 287–298 (2011)
7. Bernardi, L., Gordin, D., Rosengårdbärlund, M., et al.: Arterial function can be obtained by noninvasive finger pressure waveform. Int. J. Cardiol. **175**(1), 169–171 (2014)
8. Pickering, T.G., Hall, J.E., Appel, L., et al.: Response to recommendations for blood pressure measurement in human and experimental animals; Part 1: blood pressure measurement in humans and miscuffing: a problem with new guidelines: addendum. Hypertension **48**(1), 686–693 (2006)
9. He, X., Goubran, R., Liu, X.P.: Secondary peak detection of PPG signal for continuous cuffless arterial blood pressure measurement. IEEE Trans. Instrum. Meas. **63**(6), 1431–1439 (2014)
10. Marques, F., Ribeiro, D., Colunas, M., et al.: A truly wearable medical device for ECG, PPG and blood pressure monitoring. IEEE Trans. Biomed. Eng (2010, submitted)
11. Bose, S.S.N., Kumar, C.S.: Improving the performance of continuous non-invasive estimation of blood pressure using ECG and PPG. In: IEEE Indicon (2015)
12. Spulak, D., Cmejla, R., Fabian, V.: Parameters for mean blood pressure estimation based on electrocardiography and photoplethysmography. In: International Conference on Applied Electronics, vol. 123, no. Suppl. 1, pp. 1–4 (2011)
13. Kachuee, M., Kiani, M.M., Mohammadzade, H., et al.: Cuff-less high-accuracy calibration-free blood pressure estimation using pulse transit time. In: IEEE International Symposium on Circuits and Systems, pp. 1006–1009. IEEE (2015)
14. Puke, S., Suzuki, T., Nakayama, K., et al.: Blood pressure estimation from pulse wave velocity measured on the chest. In: International Conference of the IEEE Engineering in Medicine & Biology Society, pp. 6107–6110 (2013)
15. Kurylyak, Y., Lamonaca, F., Grimaldi, D.: A neural network-based method for continuous blood pressure estimation from a PPG signal. IEEE Instrum. Meas. Technol. Conf. **80**(11), 280–283 (2013)
16. O'Rourke, M.F.: Time domain analysis of the arterial pulse in clinical medicine. Med. Biol. Eng. Comput. **47**(2), 119–129 (2009)
17. Yan, Y.S., Zhang, Y.T.: Noninvasive estimation of blood pressure using photoplethysmographic signals in the period domain. In: Proceedings of 27th Annual International Conference of the Engineering in Medicine and Biology Society (IEEE-EMBS 2005), pp. 3583–3584 (2005)
18. Nitzan, M., Patron, A., Glik, Z., et al.: Automatic noninvasive measurement of systolic blood pressure using photoplethysmography. BioMed. Eng. OnLine **8**(1), 1–8 (2009)
19. Laurent, C., Jonsson, B., Vegfors, M., et al.: Noninvasive monitoring of systolic blood pressure on the arm utilizing photoplethysmography (PPG): clinical report. In: Biomedical Optics. International Society for Optics and Photonics, pp. 99–107 (2004)
20. Li, Z-J., Wang, C., Zhu, H., Jin, F., Ma, J-L.: The research progress of non-invasive and continuous blood pressure measurement based on photoplethysmography. Chin. J. Biomed. Eng. **31**(4), 607–614 (2012)
21. Yao, R., Zhang, Y., Chen, L., et al.: Identification of parameters of blood pressure measurement based on pulse wave. Med. Health Equip. **37**(1), 5–7 (2016)
22. Lu, H., Yan, Z., Lu, W.: A noninvasive and continuous method for blood pressure measurement using pulse wave. Chin. J. Med. Instrum. (Zhongguo yi liao qi xie za zhi) **35**(35), 169–173 (2011)
23. Mills, A.K.: Device and method for noninvasive continuous determination of physiologic characteristics. US, US6921367[P] (2005)

A Networked and Intelligent Regional Collaborative Treatment System for AMI

Ming Sheng[1(✉)], Jianwei Liu[1(✉)], Hongxia Liu[1(✉)], Yong Zhang[1(✉)],
Chunxiao Xing[1(✉)], and Yinan Li[2(✉)]

[1] Tsinghua National Laboratory for Information Science and Technology,
Department of Computer Science and Technology, Research Institute of Information Technology,
Tsinghua University, Beijing, China
{shengming,liujianwei,zhangyong05,xingcx}@tsinghua.edu.cn,
panny_lhx@163.com
[2] Yellow River Engineering Consulting Co., Ltd., Beijing 100084, China
liyinan85@gmail.com

Abstract. In "China Cardiovascular Disease Report 2015", research shows that mortality of Acute Myocardial Infarction (AMI) was rapidly increased since 2005. The mortality in 2014 was 123.92/lakh, which was 4.4 times higher than in 2002. Cardiovascular disease is ranked No. 1 in cause of death in China right now, in both rural and urban areas. This paper presents a medical information sharing platform based on mobile Internet, cloud computing and big data mining. It is designed to support the PB-level data management and analysis, and millions of concurrent instant messaging. The platform has the following functions: intelligent transportation decision support based on FMC-D time, built-in medical communication unit, built-in medical information sharing unit and quality control system of PCI hospital interventional images. The platform is divided into two parts - medical unit terminals (including EMS terminal, non-PCI hospital terminal and PCI hospital terminal) and cloud computing server, in which data is exchanged via 3G/4G wireless networks. The system has the following characteristics: (1) Timeline, which is a collection of key nodes that describe the AMI patient care process, (2) Smart recommendation technology, for example recommending hospitals based on the distance, medical care ability, idle resource. (3) Capacity to support, such as large number of concurrent collaborative treatment process among multiple PCI hospitals, multi-non-PCI medical institutions, and multi-EMS institutions, as well as the PB level data which are generated in the process.

Keywords: PCI hospital · STEMI · AMI · FMC-D time · Data analysis · Smart health

© Springer International Publishing AG 2017
C. Xing et al. (Eds.): ICSH 2016, LNCS 10219, pp. 132–143, 2017.
DOI: 10.1007/978-3-319-59858-1_13

1 Introduction

1.1 Background

The incidence of acute myocardial infarction (AMI) in China is increasing year by year and the age of victims tends to be younger. Acute ST-segment elevation myocardial infarction (STEMI) has a high mortality. Timely and accurate diagnosis and early direct PCI treatment is the key to reduce the acute phase morbidity, improve the long-term prognosis [1]. As the development of the Internet of things and mobile Internet, wearable devices and mobile smart health service have become a hot topic in recent years [2–4], which have the natural advantages in the field of health monitoring [5]. They can monitor the patients' health and motion conditions whenever and wherever possible [6–8]. With the increasing of the population of the AMI, the needs of wearable health monitoring devices increase quickly [9, 10].

In 2013, AHA "The treatment guidelines for acute ST-segment elevation myocardial infarction" [1], introduced the concept of First Medical Contact to Device (FMC-D) time, which refers to a period from the first time medical contact with STEMI patients (no distinction between medical units or level) to the time that patients in the catheter room to open the vessel (reperfusion start). In 2015, "China ST-segment elevation acute myocardial infarction diagnosis and treatment guidelines" proposes: FMC-D target time less than 90 min for the patients receiving direct PCI, and FMC-D target time less than 120 min for the patients receiving transport PCI. The concept of FMC-D emphasizes the role of pre-hospital care in the treatment of myocardial infarction, shifting the beginning of the treatment of myocardial infarction from the "first aid in hospital" to "pre-hospital care." The guidelines also suggest that FMC-D time is not only an evaluation indicator of STEMI patient treatment, but also a decision-making indicator of STEMI referral strategies. However, there are many factors that influence the FMC-D time. In the existing emergency situations, EMS, non-PCI medical institutions and the PCI hospital within the radius of treatment cannot form a unified whole. And therefore the determine of FMC-D time is lack of objective scientific basis. Therefore, the optimal selection of STEMI patient referral and revascularization strategy cannot be achieved. Regional collaborative treatment system can effectively integrate the existing medical resources by combining a number of PCI hospitals, EMS, and non-PCI medical institutions within a certain distance range into a regional centralized coordination treatment system. The system does the overall coordination and shortens the rescue radius and the time to develop the most effective treatment strategy for each STEMI patient in the shortest space-time distance.

1.2 Technology Reviews

Despite years of efforts in shorten the time of FMC-D in AMI treatment, effective solutions could be summarized into the following two types:

1. Multi-centers regional collaborative treatment systems, such as Lifeline program [1], in which 1500 pre-hospitals first aid systems and 450 hospitals in 17 US cities are divided into 5 regional systems. In each regional system, medical institutions within

the scope are integrated into a single STEMI treatment center, and thus aiming to enhance the capability of each institution in the treatment of AMI either by adopting collective wisdoms of advanced treatment procedure or by following an adjusted standard procedure protocol signed by all institutions according to individual differences.

2. Linear regional collaborative treatment systems based on single PCI or Chest Pain Center, in which medical institutions within a certain distance of the center are integrated into a treatment system.

The main drawbacks of the above solutions are the following:

1. There are many communication modes in treatment regional. It is difficult to be unified coordinated and the information flow ability is poor.
2. FMC-D time is used as a decision indicator for revascularization strategy. Pre-hospital assessment mainly depends on experience of EMS staff, which is lack of objective, and intelligent decision support.
3. Radiation range is small. The number of people who benefit from the system is limited. The scope of the medical unit interaction with the outside is poor. As a result, it cannot form a complementary advantage or resources.

The advantages and disadvantages of the current emergency systems are shown in the following Table 1.

Table 1. List of current emergency systems

System	Drawbacks
Bian Que fly save	Lack of data analysis, mining and related decision support, a common emergency platform
Pre-hospital care networking program	Lack of inter-regional collaboration among multiple hospitals, lack of data mining and analysis, a common emergency platform
Intelligent emergency monitoring system	Lack of inter-regional collaboration among multiple hospitals, lack of data mining and analysis, a common emergency platform
Interconnection first aid APP	Lack of inter-regional collaboration among multiple hospitals, lack of data mining, data analysis and lack of expert guidance, a common emergency platform

1.3 Purpose

To solve the above problems, we aim to provide a medical information sharing platform based on mobile internet and cloud computing technology, and establish a networked and intelligent regional collaborative treatment system for acute myocardial infarction, which is shorted for "RCTS-AMI".

Specifically, this paper provides a medical information sharing platform based on mobile internet and cloud computing technology, which has the following major functions: Intelligent Transport Decision Support Based on FMC-D Time, communication of medical units in the system, information sharing of medical units within the system and PCI hospital interventional image quality control management. The system is divided into two parts. They are medical unit terminal (including EMS terminal, non-PCI hospital terminal and PCI hospital terminal) and cloud computing server. It uses 3G/4G wireless network for data exchange. In ambulance client takes into account the user's operating experience, and develop a system based on the Android. Cloud computing server processing center is deployed on the cloud server, according to the concept of SOA architecture framework for the design, based on the data warehouse for business data depth mining analysis.

The features of this system include:

1. The framework is based on timeline. Timeline is a collection of key nodes that describe the AMI patient care process, such as calling the EMS time, EMS response time, ambulance arrival time, first chest pain episode time, the chest pain onset time, EMS first ECG time, and so on. Through the statistics of the key event time node, the rational allocation of resources, auxiliary decision support and other methods, we can improve the treatment efficiency of AMI. Timeline is shown in Fig. 1.

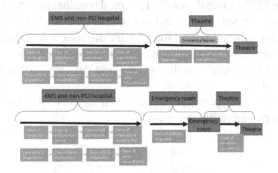

Fig. 1. Timeline of RCTS-AMI

2. Smart recommendation technology. (1) Real-time hospital medical resources information (such as availability of beds, doctors and surgical equipments), (2) Geographic location information, which mainly balances the road congestion and the distance from the target hospital information, (3) Treatment capacity, which mainly refers to the PCI hospital treatment capacity through the mining and analysis of the historical data.

3. Large-scale support. In ambulance, the client terminal takes into account the user's operating experience and develops a system based on the Android. Cloud computing server processing center is deployed on the cloud server, according to the concept of SOA architecture and the XMPP (Jabber) protocol communication mechanism based on the concept of open source framework for the design, based on the data warehouse for business data depth mining analysis. Applications in Beijing and other places shows that the system supports PCI hospitals in the region, multi-non-PCI medical institutions, multi-EMS institutions concurrent collaborative treatment

process and the PB data generated in the process. In a complete, independent RCTS-AMI system, it supports 500–800 PCI hospitals and non-PCI hospitals, 1 million–2 million terminals, 2000–2500 doctors.

This paper is organized as follows. The second section mainly introduces the related methods. The third section displays the key technologies. The fourth section is the application and analysis of the system. The last section summarize the paper.

2 System Structure Design

2.1 The Overall Design Framework

The main purpose of the platform is that the patients could get to the regional PCI hospital or chest pain center and successfully completed STEMI treatment as soon as possible. The platform is designed into following functions: Intelligent Transport Decision Support Based on FMC-D Time, communication of medical units in the system, information sharing of medical units within the system and PCI hospital interventional image quality control management. The system is divided into two parts. They are medical unit terminal (including EMS terminal, non-PCI hospital terminal and PCI hospital terminal) and cloud computing server. It uses 3G/4G wireless network for data exchange. In ambulance the client terminal takes into account the user's operating experience and implemented in Android. Cloud computing server processing center is deployed on the cloud. We use SOA framework for the system, and data warehouse for business data depth mining analysis.

As shown in Fig. 2, this platform has achieved the STEMI patient networked and intelligent regional collaborative treatment.

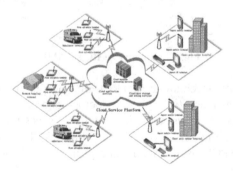

Fig. 2. Topology architecture of RCTS-AMI

The core of the platform is the cloud server. The architecture of it is based on Huading, which is a general big data management and analysis system based on the Hadoop and Spark ecosystem developed in Tsinghua University. Huading also integrates the column database, memory database and other modules. The platform can efficiently manage PB level data, including structured, semi-structured, unstructured data, and provide support for relevant analysis and mining. The RCTS_AMI introduced in this paper is deployed on the Huading cloud platform, realizes the management and analysis of large data. At the same time, Huading cloud efficient distributed file system and database cluster provides support for the actual business of large-scale remote consultation, instant messaging, message push, and data transmission. For remote consultation, instant messaging and related messaging, the platform mainly uses the communication mechanism based on XMPP (Jabber) protocol. For data sharing and other operations, according to the size of the data, the platform uses HTTP protocol, FTP transmission and other models to deal with.

From the specific business process, the doctors can use different ambulance terminal, different network hospitals to upload their own data to launch remote consultation. With the help of cloud platform for a unified calculation of the various resources (mainly the doctors resources and surgical resources of chest pain center hospital, real-time road resources, etc.), the patient's consultation information will be sent to the optimal chest pain center hospital, a series of remote consultation and may require PCI treatment.

As long as the patient enters into the collaborative treatment system, including community hospitals, network hospitals, emergency vehicles, emergency, etc., they can obtain the treatment in the chest pain center hospital who join the platform network according to their characteristics.

According to the coordinated deployment of all joined the chest pain center hospital resources, the system can help the patients to find the optimal treatment channel.

The system architecture is shown in Fig. 3. The data sources include EMS terminal, PCI hospital terminal and HIS system, non-PCI hospital terminal and HIS system, and traffic implementation data. The functional units include FMC-D intelligent transportation decision support system, medical unit communication system, medical information sharing system, and PCI hospital intervention image quality control system. User oriented features include EMS, non PCI institutions, PCI hospitals and related medical regulatory agencies. The ultimate realization of the functions mainly include the optimal transport decision-making, high efficiency first aid, intelligent two-way consultation, regional system quality control. In general, it is reasonable to analyze and mobilize all emergency resources to achieve the purpose of efficient treatment.

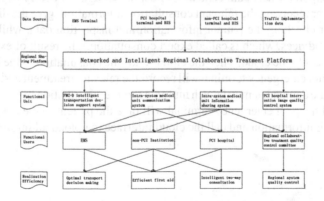

Fig. 3. System architecture of RCTS-AMI

2.2 Intelligent Transportation Decision Support Based on FMC-D Time

When several PCI hospital or chest pain centers form a regional coalition, the medical institutions in the radius of STEMI patients will form a group through the network platform, the platform will use the cloud computing technology to provide intelligent decision support for the patient transport treatment strategy.

2.3 Communication of Medical Units in the System

In the regional collaborative treatment system, EMS, non-PCI medical institutions and a number of PCI hospitals or chest pain center will achieve medical communications through mobile Internet technology, including remote consultation and real-time monitoring. Through medical collecting equipment which support Bluetooth 4 protocol, the terminal can communicate with multiple devices, and monitor the patient's vital signs and symptoms (including blood oxygen, blood pressure, ECG, blood indicators and other medical data) in real time. For the collected data, we use 3G/4G wireless network and a persistent connection to ensure low power consumption, low flow consumption. The system realizes high concurrent real-time message push and remote real-time communication, so that other medical units can catch the progress of the disease, and prepare in advance. The communication platform can achieve the pre-hospital information transmission, and improve the treatment efficiency of STEMI.

The communication between the medical units in the system mainly includes three parts: EMS/non-PCI hospital emergency terminal, cloud computing server, and chest pain center/PCI hospital experts. EMS/non-PCI hospital emergency terminal launches remote consultation. The terminal can record the patient's information and vital signs. Then we start the real-time communication and data transmission system, which can be applied for remote consultation. The implementation of the interface of instant messaging, data transmission systems and remote consultation information are in the clouds. The cloud will receive relevant information from the EMS/non-PCI hospital emergency terminal at the same time, store them and then push to the chest pain center/ PCI hospital experts. Chest pain center/PCI hospital experts will carry out the relevant admissions after receiving the relevant consultation information, give the diagnosis and treatment after checking the patient information and inspection data, while providing PCI treatment advices, which is called expert consultation. The result of expert consultation will be sent to the cloud. Then the cloud sends the consultation to the EMS. EMS/ non-PCI hospital emergency terminal will record the relevant treatment and medication. According to the demand, it may launch multiple remote consultation processes. Finally, EMS/non-PCI hospital emergency terminal will take the patient to the hospital, record the transferring information and call the cloud interface to upload all information to the cloud (Fig. 4).

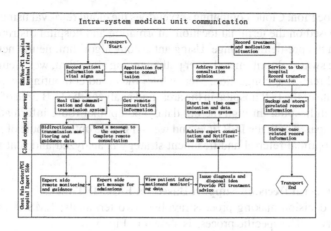

Fig. 4. Intra-system medical unit communication

2.4 Design of Intelligent Referral Decision Support Based on FMC-D Time

EMS decision-supporting process mainly involves two parts: EMS terminal and cloud computing server.

In the EMS terminal, the current location information can be obtained based on real-time GPS positioning system. The terminal sends the relevant location information to the cloud. The cloud receives the location information from EMS terminal, and generates the optimal route, which is based on the locations of the PCI hospitals and real-time traffic path. It also considers the hospital STEMI treatment D-B time, which is used as an important weight parameter in the optimal route. Finally, the calculated results (including hospital information and routes) are sent to the EMS terminal, which completes the whole process of the optimal route selection.

3   Key Technologies

3.1 Smart Recommendation

Smart recommendations are based on the following information: (1) Real-time hospital medical resources information, such as bed resources, doctor resources, surgical resources, etc., (2) Geographical location information, mainly is used to calculate the road congestion and distance from the target hospital, (3) Treatment capacity, mainly refers to the measurement of PCI hospital treatment capacity through mining and analysis the history data generated in the treatment process. There are two kinds of intelligent recommendations: 1. Intelligent Transportation Decision Support based on FMC-D time, 2. Intelligent Referral Decision Support Based on FMC-D Time.

Intelligent Transportation Decision Support Based on FMC-D Time
EMS terminal generates positioning basis through the GPS satellite positioning system and mobile base station signal, and then sends the information to the location server to

calculate the location. Cloud computing server does the cloud retrieval using LBS cloud technology, based on the terminal location information and hospital distribution information within the pre-defined range. Using ant colony algorithm, neural network algorithm, particle swarm algorithm and other path planning algorithm, we calculate the best route to avoid real-time congestion. Meanwhile, the cloud computing server retrieves the medical data of the PCI hospital in the area, and analyzes the D-B time of the STEMI patients in each hospital through the big data. The optimal route information to each hospital is compared with the D-B time, and we can get the optimal route of pre-hospital FMC-D. The optimal referral and treatment strategy is analyzed and sent to the EMS terminal.

Intelligent Referral Decision Support Based on FMC-D Time

EMS referral decision-making process involves two terminals: EMS terminal, cloud computing server. The specific process is shown in Fig. 5.

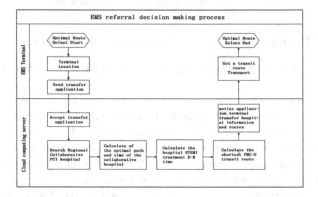

Fig. 5. EMS Referral Decision Support process

In addition to the optimal path selection based on GIS, RCTS-AMI can also calculate the hospital STEMI treatment D-B time. The result used as an important weight parameter of the whole optimal path, and then calculate the shortest path of FMC-D time. Finally, the calculated results (including hospital information and routes) are sent to the EMS terminal in the form of message push, which completes the whole process of the optimal route selection.

3.2 Large-Scale Rapid Response

In the treatment process, there is a large number of transmission and reception of concurrent remote consultation. There is also a concurrent peer to peer instant messaging. At the same time, the remote consultation will also transfer large files, such as audio and video images. In order to solve the above problems, we designed a communication mechanism that integrates XMPP (Jabber) protocol, HTTPS and FTP protocol to support the remote consultation and instant messaging needed in the treatment process. For data sharing and other operations, according to the size of the data, the platform uses HTTP protocol, FTP transmission and other models to deal with (Fig. 6).

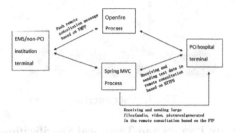

Fig. 6. Communication mechanism

In the remote consultation, the message pushing and the instant messaging are realized based on the XMPP protocol. The text data involved in the remote consultation are transmitted based on the HTTPS protocol. The large files (including audio, video, pictures) involved in the remote consultation are transmitted based on the FTP protocol. HTTPS and FTP are used to implement the functions of the server terminal based on springMVC.

4   Application and Analysis

4.1   Application, Design and Development

The RCTS_AMI system has been deployed in the western region of Beijing, and integrated with the EMS system in western Beijing, 13 chest pain center hospitals and many non-PCI medical institutions, to establish STEMI collaborative treatment network. Through GPS positioning, cloud computing of real time road traffic data and PCI data, so that any STEMI patient into the treatment network can get the optimal treatment approach, bid farewell to the treatment mode that fighting themself in the major hospitals. At the same time the system has also been deployed in Jinzhou, and there are four PCI hospitals in the Jinzhou system.

The RCTS_AMI was developed using Android SDK, Python and Java, and connected to devices via Bluetooth or wireless technology. The Fig. 7 shows an example of the user interface.

4.2   Analysis

The Effect of Regional Coordinated Treatment on the Prognosis of Patients
RCTS_AMI contains a number of PCI hospitals as the center of regional collaborative treatment network. Without changing the existing emergency resource allocation pattern, through the network, RCTS_AMI builds an intelligent platform for non-PCI hospital STEMI patients whom can be transferred into PCI hospitals and receive the treatment, which can shorten the treatment time and improve the success rate.

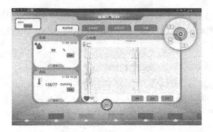

Fig. 7. User interface

Intra-regional Treatment Process and Technical Specifications
Through the practice of RCTS_AMI, we establish and improve the regional cooperation process and technical specifications of the STEMI patients. The process and technical specifications and other mature experience can be promoted to further and even national, so that more areas can achieve synergistic treatment of STEMI patients in the region.

Intra-regional PCI and non-PCI Hospitals
Through RCTS_AMI, PCI hospitals in the regional collaborative treatment network not only build the hospital green channel as the goal, and wait for the arrival of patients, but further links pre-hospital cares and primary non-PCI hospitals for more STEMI patients. In the medical system, we really shorten the time delay, which means to shorten the time of FMC-D. At the same time, the system can exchange information with other PCI hospitals in the regional to improve the ability of diagnosis and treatment of STEMI.

STEMI Regional Collaborative Treatment Network
Through RCTS_AMI, it is possible to establish STEMI process and norm of the regional collaborative treatment network, form STEMI regional collaborative standard treatment processes and industry norms. Further we can reach a consensus on promoting the domestic STEMI regional consensus treatment.

Reducing the Cost of Emergency Care for AMI
RCTS_AMI improves the STEMI treatment efficiency, reduces morbidity and the national and individual health expenditure, and produces higher social economic benefits.

Good Prospect of Application
Through RCTS_AMI, the establishment of STEMI regional collaborative treatment network can fill the domestic gaps in the treatment of STEMI patients, which can significantly improve the level of linkage between emergency care system and hospital system, which follows the international trend. The experiences and methods can be promoted to other areas and even national. By ensuring the medical effect of patients, the system improves the treatment efficiency, and has a considerable application prospects.

5   Summary

This paper presents a medical information sharing platform based on mobile Internet, cloud computing and big data mining. It is capable to manage PB-level data, and support millions of concurrent instant messaging. The platform has the following functions: FMC-D time based intelligent transport decision support, medical unit communication in the system, medical unit information sharing and PCI hospital interventional image quality control management. The system is divided into two parts. They are medical unit terminals (including EMS terminal, non-PCI hospital terminal and PCI hospital terminal) and cloud computing server. The system uses 3G/4G wireless network for data exchange. The system has the following characteristics: (1) The architecture designed around the time axis. Timeline is a collection of key nodes that describe the AMI patient care process, (2) Intelligent recommended technology, such as recommending hospitals based on the distance, medical care ability, idle resource and so on. (3) Large-scale support. The practice in Beijing and other places shows that the system has support for multiple PCI hospitals in the region, Multi-non-PCI medical institutions, multi-EMS institutions concurrent collaborative treatment process.

Acknowledgment. This work was supported by NSFC (91646202), the National High-tech R&D Program of China (Grant No. SS2015AA020102), the 1000-Talent program, Tsinghua University Initiative Scientific Research Program.

References

1. Warren, S., Craft, R., Bosma, B.: Designing smart health care technology into the home of the future. In: Workshops on Future Medical Devices, vol. 2, p. 667 (1999)
2. Fox, S., Rainie, L.: Vital decisions: how internet users decide what information to trust when they or their loved ones are sick: plus a guide from the medical library association about smart health-search strategies and good web sites. Pew Internet & American Life Project (2002)
3. Clancy, M.: Getting to 'smart' health care. Health Aff. 25(6), w589–w592 (2006)
4. Lymberis, A.: Research and development of smart wearable health applications: the challenge ahead. Stud. Health Technol. Inform. 108, 155–161 (2004)
5. Irwig, L.: "Smart health choices," Judy Irwig (2007)
6. Kao, H.-Y., Cheng, Y.-T., Chien, Y.-K.: Develop and evaluate the mobile-based self-management application for tele-healthcare service. In: Ali, M., Pan, J.-S., Chen, S.-M., Horng, M.-F. (eds.) IEA/AIE 2014. LNCS, vol. 8481, pp. 460–469. Springer, Cham (2014). doi: 10.1007/978-3-319-07455-9_48
7. Elgazzar, K., AboElFotoh, M., Martin, P., Hassanein, H.S.: Ubiquitous health monitoring using mobile web services. In: ANT/MobiWIS, pp. 332–339 (2012)
8. García-Sánchez, P., González, J., Miguel Mora, A., Prieto, A.: Deploying intelligent E-health services in a mobile gateway. Expert Syst. 40(4), 1231–1239 (2013)
9. Deng, Z., Mo, X., Liu, S.: Comparison of the middle-aged and older users' adoption of mobile smart health services in China. Int. J. Med. Inform. 83(3), 210–224 (2014)

Medical Monitoring and Information Extraction, Clinical and Medical Data Mining

AZPharm MetaAlert: A Meta-learning Framework for Pharmacovigilance

Xiao Liu[1(✉)] and Hsinchun Chen[2]

[1] Department of Operations and Information Systems, University of Utah, Salt Lake City, USA
xiao.liu@eccles.utah.edu
[2] Department of Management Information Systems, University of Arizona, Tucson, USA
hchen@eller.arizona.edu

Abstract. Pharmacovigilance is the research related to the detection, assessment, understanding, and prevention of adverse drug events. Despite the research efforts in pharmacovigilance in recent year, current approaches are insufficient in detecting adverse drug reaction (ADR) signals timely across different datasets. In this study, we develop an integrated and high-performance AZ Pharm Meta-Alert framework for efficient and accurate post-approval pharmacovigilance. Our approach extracts adverse drug events from patient social media, electronic health records, and FDA's Adverse Event Reporting System (FAERS) and integrates ADR signals with stacking and bagging methods. Experiment results show that our approach achieves 71% in precision, 90% in recall, and 80% in f-measure for ADR signal detection and significantly outperforms the traditional signal detection methods.

Keywords: Pharmacovigilance · Adverse drug event · Meta-learning · Deep-learning · Drug safety surveillance

1 Introduction

Pharmacovigilance (PhV), also referred to as drug safety surveillance, has been defined as "the science and activities related to the detection, assessment, understanding and prevention of adverse drug events (ADEs)." An adverse drug event (ADE) can be any unfavorable and unintended sign, symptom, disease, or death temporally associated with the use of a drug, irrespective of whether it is considered to be caused by this drug or not. An adverse drug reaction (ADR) indicates a causal effect between a drug and an adverse event.

Pharmacovigilance research has steadily grown in the past decade via different approaches. Drug regulatory agencies (e.g., FDA and WHO) have developed spontaneous reporting systems (SRS) to collect reports of suspected adverse drug events (ADEs) from health professionals, consumers, and pharmaceutical companies. The secondary analyses of electronic health records (EHRs) and administrative claims from hospital information systems also hold the promise of new evidence for adverse drug events. The public availability of chemical and biological knowledge bases opens new opportunity to study molecular perspectives of adverse drug events. Patients'

© Springer International Publishing AG 2017
C. Xing et al. (Eds.): ICSH 2016, LNCS 10219, pp. 147–154, 2017.
DOI: 10.1007/978-3-319-59858-1_14

discussions about treatments on social networks and forums become another emerging source for adverse drug reaction detection.

Despite the efforts in improving post-approval pharmacovigilance, current approaches are still not sufficient. Only half of newly discovered serious ADRs are detected within seven years of drug approval [1]. The reason for the delay in ADR detection is two-fold. First, the performance of ADR detection is subjected to adverse drug event report coverage. Most adverse drug events are not reported timely to support drug safety decision-making. The reporting rate of adverse drug events to drug regulatory agencies is lower than 10% [2]. Second, ADR detection is limited by the accuracy of signal detection algorithms. No single ADR signal detection method has emerged as a state-of-the-art technique for detecting ADR signals.

Due to these limitations, there is a need for pharmacovigilance research to move toward integrated analysis with multiple healthcare data sources. In this study, we seek to develop an integrated and high-performance AZPharm MetaAlert framework for efficient and accurate post-approval pharmacovigilance.

2   Related Work

ADR signal detection process aims to highlight significant associations (signals) between drugs and adverse events in data. Based on these associations, drug safety regulation agencies can initiate regulatory actions or in-depth investigations. Various signal detection methods have been developed. These signal detection methods can be categorized into three approaches. Disproportionality analysis (DPA) approach searches the data set for 'interesting' associations using two-dimensional contingency table and ranks the associations in order of 'interestingness.' This approach has been applied to different data sources: spontaneous reports [3]; electronic health records (EHRs) [4]; and patient social media [1].

Logistic regression approach is popular in pharmacovigilance due to its ability to control the presence of other co-medications, co-morbidities, and confounding indications. Bayesian logistic regression classification method was used to identify ADRs in WHO's VigiBase [5]. Shrinkage logistic regression is used to identify ADRs from lab tests and discharge summaries in EHRs [6]. Ordinal logistic regression was adopted to predict adverse events based on the data from PubChem and Canadian Adverse Drug Reaction Databases [7].

Unsupervised machine learning methods such as association rule mining and bi-clustering have been adopted to find associations between drugs and adverse events. Association rule mining can discover drug-adverse event associations in both spontaneous reports [6, 8]; and patient social media [1]. However, no single signal detection method has significantly outperformed the others.

Many researchers believe that combining drug safety information across different data sources may potentially improve the performance. Recent studies have developed several preliminary signal combination strategies. Harpaz et al. [6] devised a voting strategy to combine signals from FAERS and EHR data. A Bayes graphic model was developed to combine signals from FAERS and EHRs [9]. These studies demonstrate the value of the signal combination. There is a need for developing an advanced signal detection model which can leverage multiple data sources and signal detection algorithms to achieve high accuracy and early detection of ADRs. We propose the following research questions:

1. How can we develop an integrated research framework for accurate and timely detection of adverse drug reactions with the clinical evidence from social media, EHR, and SRSs?
2. How can we leverage multiple sources of adverse drug events to improve the performance of adverse drug reaction signal detection?
3. How can we develop a combined model with various signal detection algorithms to improve the performance of adverse drug reaction signal detection?

3 Research Design

To address these questions, we propose the AZPharm MetaAlert research framework for integrated pharmacovigilance as illustrated in Fig. 1. Major components are explained in detail below.

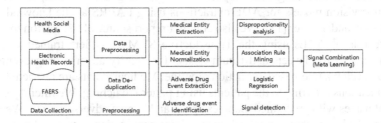

Fig. 1. AZPharm MetaAlert framework for integrated pharmacovigilance

3.1 Data Collection

Our health social media data come from American Diabetes Association (ADA) online community, and Twitter, a micro-blog social platform. From Feb. 2009 to Sept. 2015, we have collected 360, 787 posts from ADA and 207, 295 original tweets related to diabetes drugs. The spontaneous drug safety reports come from FDA's Adverse Event Reporting System. From Jan. 2004 to Aug. 2015, we identified 102, 358 reports related to diabetes drugs from FAERS for analysis. We obtain EHRs of diabetes patients in a 600-bed hospital in Taiwan from Nov. 2003 to Apr. 2012. Both structured and unstructured electronic healthcare data are included in this study. In total, we obtained 26, 714 clinical documents from 13, 109 diabetes patients.

3.2 Preprocessing

To preprocess the health social media content, we develop a text cleaning process to remove URLs, duplicate punctuation, and personally identifiable information. We conduct sentence boundary detection, and tokenization on posts from Twitter and the ADA online community, and clinical documents in EHR data. We remove duplicated reports in FAERS by verifying the demographic data and co-medications. Reports that share more than 12 attributes in common are considered duplicated and removed [6].

3.3 Adverse Drug Event Identification

To identify medical events and drug names from health social media and clinical documents in EHR, we first automatically label drug entities and medical events in social media and clinical notes with the UMLS, CHV, and FAERS lexicons [10]. To identify consumer vocabularies and named entities with typos, we extend the medical entity extraction with Long-Short Term Memory (LSTM) network[1]. LSTM network is the state-of-the-art deep learning based entity extraction model [12]. Embeddings of all the words in a sentence are the input sequence; entity types of these words are the output of the model. We standardize drug name entities to their generic names with RxNorm[2]. Medical events described by both healthcare professionals and consumers domestic and abroad. For medical event normalization, we match the terms with the Consumer Health Vocabulary[3] to normalize them to standard medical terms.

To extract adverse drug event reports from patient-generated data, we train two distant supervision models for ADE extractions using FAERS as the knowledge base for the forum, and Twitter [11]. We also conduct report source classification to identify patient reports of ADEs using the Transductive SVM classifier[4] trained with 1000 labeled instances for Tweets and forum posts. To identify adverse drug events from EHR, we develop a rule-based extraction pipeline. Medical events are restricted to only positive mentions referring to the patients using pattern matching. We filter drug names and event names with predefined diabetes drugs and known adverse events. We extract drug prescribed, symptoms, medical events from each patient's medical records and order them by their timestamps. Any adverse symptoms and events following a drug prescription are possible adverse drug events. Drug indications (the reason a drug is prescribed) and drug interactions are removed to avoid confounding.

3.4 Signal Detection and Combination

We develop a meta-learning approach for ADR signal detection with stacking and bagging methods. Figure 2 illustrates the detailed process. Our single method signal detection incorporates an array of drug safety data mining methods including disproportionality analysis (DPA) such as reporting ratio (RR), proportional reporting ratio (PRR), reporting odds ratio (ROR), and information component (IC), shrinkage logistic regression (Lasso regression), and association rule mining. These methods are applied to each data source resulting in 18 result sets for ADR signals.

---

[1] https://www.tensorflow.org/versions/r0.9/tutorials/recurrent/index.html.

[2] https://www.nlm.nih.gov/research/umls/rxnorm/.

[3] http://consumerhealthvocab.chpc.utah.edu/CHVwiki/.

[4] http://svmlight.joachims.org/.

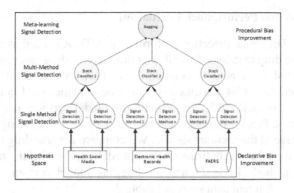

Fig. 2. Meta-learning approach for ADR signal detection

Stacking method combines multiple learning algorithms in parallel for performance boosting. We use stacking method over other meta-learning methods because stacking methods can capture the variance in the results of different learning algorithms and enhance the performance with the variance. We develop a bagging strategy to exploit the variation in data [13]. Social media and EHR data have a smaller quantity of reports but are more sensitive to new and unique events. Bagging can preserve the signals from spontaneous reports without masking new and unique events in social media and EHR. Both bagging and stacking classifiers utilize the random forest classification algorithms to aggregate the results from the lower levels.

4   Experiments

4.1   Medical Entity Extraction Evaluation

Medical entity extraction is conducted and evaluated on three data sources: patient forum (ADA online community), Twitter, and clinical notes in EHR. Drug names and medical events from 500 forum posts, 1000 tweets, and 200 clinical notes are annotated as a gold standard to evaluate medical entity extraction performance. The evaluation results are shown in Table 1. Deep learning methods outperformed lexicon-based approach in social media data. The lexicon-based approach still performs better in medical entity extraction from clinical notes.

Table 1. Medical entity extraction results

Data	Approach	Drug			Medical Event		
		Preision	Recall	F-measure	Preision	Recall	F-measure
Forum	Lexicon-based	94.3%	81.4%	87.4%	86.30%	78.7%	82.3%
	LSTM+lexicon	92.3%	87.6%	**89.9%**	83.60%	85.0%	**84.3%**
Twitter	Lexicon-based	90.4%	76.8%	83.0%	80.50%	73.5%	76.8%
	LSTM+lexicon	86.0%	84.1%	**85.0%**	77.10%	79.6%	**78.3%**
Clinical notes	Lexicon-based	84.0%	84.2%	84.1%	90.60%	88.6%	89.6%
	LSTM+lexicon	82.0%	79.7%	80.8%	86.10%	84.2%	85.1%

4.2 Signal Detection Performance Evaluation

To evaluate the ADR signal detection performance, SIDER is used as a gold standard dataset for adverse drug reactions. SIDER contains adverse drug reactions for marketed medicines extracted from public documents and package inserts. There are 6,192 adverse drug reactions for 74 diabetes drugs in generic names (124 in brand name) in SIDER released from Oct. 2015. We evaluate the model performance with precision and recall measures. Precision reflects the accuracy of the detected signals and recall reflects the coverage of the accurate signals. We compare adverse drug reaction signals predicted by our model with confirmed ADRs in SIDER, the stacking model performance with each method (Table 2), and the bagging model performance with three stacking models on different data sources (Table 3).

Table 2. Signal detection methods and stacking performance

Method	Social Media			EHR			FAERS		
	Precision	Recall	F-measure	Precision	Recall	F-measure	Precision	Recall	F-measure
RR	66.9%	12.0%	20.3%	45.7%	28.5%	35.1%	35.1%	83.9%	49.5%
PRR	71.5%	9.9%	17.4%	67.9%	25.2%	36.8%	38.5%	81.9%	52.4%
ROR	62.0%	10.5%	18.0%	72.1%	29.6%	42.0%	38.9%	74.3%	51.1%
IC	66.9%	12.0%	20.3%	75.1%	28.6%	41.4%	36.8%	82.2%	50.8%
LR	67.6%	17.5%	27.8%	79.3%	30.3%	43.8%	44.4%	86.0%	58.6%
ARM	68.4%	14.8%	24.3%	68.9%	30.1%	41.9%	37.0%	75.1%	49.6%
Stacking	73.5%	17.8%	28.7%	80.0%	32.8%	46.5%	45.0%	86.0%	59.1%

Table 3. Bagging performance compared to stacking results.

Data	Precision	Recall	F-measure
Social Media	73.5%	17.8%	28.7%
EHR	80.0%	32.8%	46.5%
FAERS	45.0%	86.0%	59.1%
All	71.0%	90.2%	79.5%

According to our experiment results, stacking the signal detection algorithms can improve the accuracy of ADR signal detection. Bagging the signal detection results from three data sets increases the recall of ADR signal detection. Adverse drug events in EHR data has resulted in the high-precision prediction of adverse drug reactions with EHR data. Social media can also provide accurate reports of adverse drug events, leading to good precision in ADR detection. As each data source contains different ADR signals, bagging method obtains a higher recall of ADR signals.

5 Discussions and Conclusion

In this study, we develop an integrated and high-performance meta-learning framework for pharmacovigilance. Our experiment results show that each signal detection method identifies different adverse drug reaction signals and their accuracy varies. We also find that each data source for pharmacovigilance has different coverage of adverse drug reaction signals.

The existence of variance in data sources and learning methods demonstrates the room for a meta-learning process to enhance the adverse drug reaction signal detection performance. Our proposed stacking method leverages the variance in current signal detection algorithm, and the bagging method leverages the variance in adverse drug event reports from multiple sources. Both strategies effectively improve the performance of adverse drug reaction signal detection.

Acknowledgement. This work was supported in part by National Science Foundation SBIR/STTR Award ID #1417181 and #1622788.

References

1. Yang, C.C., Yang, H., Jiang, L.: Postmarketing drug safety surveillance using publicly available health-consumer-contributed content in social media. ACM Trans. Manag. Inf. Syst. (TMIS) **5**(1), 2 (2014)
2. Leaman, R., Wojtulewicz, L., Sullivan, R., Skariah, A., Yang, J., Gonzalez G.: Towards internet-age pharmacovigilance: extracting adverse drug reactions from user posts to health-related social networks. In: Proceedings of the Workshop on Biomedical Natural Language Processing, Uppsala, pp. 117–125 (2010)
3. Vilar, S., Harpaz, R., Chase, H.S., Costanzi, S., Rabadan, R., Friedman, C.: Facilitating adverse drug event detecting in pharmacovigilance databases using molecular structure similarity: application to rhadomyolysis. J. Am. Med. Inform. Assoc. **18**(suppl. 1), i73–i80 (2011)
4. Zorych, I., Madigan, D., Ryan, P., Bate, A.: Disproportionality methods for pharmacovigilance in longitude observational database. Stat. Methods Med. Res. **22**(1), 39–56 (2011)
5. Caster, O., Noren, G.N., Madigan, D., Bate, A.: Large-scale regression-based pattern discovery: the example of screening the WHO global drug safety database. Stat. Anal. Data Min. **3**, 197–208 (2010)
6. Harpaz, R., Vilar, S., DuMouchel, W., Salmasian, H., Haerian, K., Shah, N.H., Friedman, C.: Combing signals from spontaneous reports and electronic health records for detection of adverse drug reactions. J. Am. Med. Inform. Assoc. **20**(3), 413–419 (2012)
7. Pouliot, Y., Chiang, A.P., Butte, A.J.: Predicting adverse drug reactions using publicly available PubChem BioAssay data. Clin. Pharmacol. Ther. **90**(1), 90–99 (2011)
8. Rouane-Hacene, M., Toussaint, Y., Valtchev, P.: Mining safety signals in spontaneous reports database using concept analysis. In: Combi, C., Shahar, Y., Abu-Hanna, A. (eds.) AIME 2009. LNCS, vol. 5651, pp. 285–294. Springer, Heidelberg (2009). doi: 10.1007/978-3-642-02976-9_41
9. Harpaz, R., DuMouchel, W., LePendu, P., Shah, N.H.: Empirical Bayes model to combine signals of adverse drug reactions. In: Proceedings of the 19th ACM SIGKDD International Conference on Knowledge Discovery and Data Mining, pp. 1339–1347. ACM, August 2013
10. Liu, X., Chen, H.: AZDrugMiner: an information extraction system for mining patient-reported adverse drug events in online patient forums. In: Zeng, D., et al. (eds.) ICSH 2013. LNCS, vol. 8040, pp. 134–150. Springer, Heidelberg (2013). doi: 10.1007/978-3-642-39844-5_16

11. Liu, X., Liu, J., Chen, H.: Identifying adverse drug events from health social media: a case study on heart disease discussion forums. In: Zheng, X., Zeng, D., Chen, H., Zhang, Y., Xing, C., Neill, D.B. (eds.) ICSH 2014. LNCS, vol. 8549, pp. 25–36. Springer, Cham (2014). doi: 10.1007/978-3-319-08416-9_3
12. Sutskever, I., Vinyals, O., Le, Q.V.: Sequence to sequence learning with neural networks. In: Advances in Neural Information Processing Systems, pp. 3104–3112 (2014)
13. Liang, G., Cohn, A.G.: An effective approach for imbalanced classification: unevenly balanced bagging. In: AAAI, June 2013

MedC: Exploring and Predicting Medicine Interactions to Support Integrative Chinese Medicine

Xin Li[✉], Haobo Gu, and Yu Tong

Department of Information Systems, City University of Hong Kong, Kowloon, Hong Kong
{Xin.Li,yutong}@cityu.edu.hk, bohgu22222-x@my.cityu.edu.hk

Abstract. Chinese medicine is increasingly being used with Western medicine in practice, especially for treatment of chronic diseases. In this integrative medicine process, it is necessary to understand the interactions between Chinese and Western medicine to reduce adverse events. However, compared to Western medicine, there are limited studies that summarize findings on Chinese medicine interactions and effectively present such findings to practitioners. Built upon the MedC literature analysis system, this paper proposes a Chinese medicine analysis and prediction framework that can effectively present Chinese medicine interactions and connect them with the clinical evidence documented in literature. The system can support Chinese medicine scholars and facilitate research on integrative Chinese medicine.

Keywords: Chinese medicine · Drug interaction · Text mining · Visualization

1 Introduction

Traditional Chinese medicine originates from the long-time practice of Chinese physicians and plays an important role in Chinese history and society. Many pioneers tested the effects of Chinese herbs and medicines and documented them in literature. In 2015, the Nobel Prize in Physiology or Medicine was awarded to YouyouTu due to her contribution to finding Artemisinin. The finding of Artemisinin was benefited from traditional Chinese medicine literature.

In recent years, Chinese medicine is increasingly being used with Western medicine in practice, especially for treating chronic diseases [1]. However, to (successfully) integrate Chinese medicine and Western medicine, it is necessary to understand the interactions among medicines. Otherwise, they may cause serious problems in clinical practice. In Western medicine, there have been intensive studies on medicine interactions, such as using biological experiments [2] to identify them. One challenge in extending studies to Chinese medicine is that a Chinese medicine usually contains several compounds, and thus its interaction would be more complicated. Furthermore, there is a need to aggregate the clinical evidence in the literature on the side effects of integrative Chinese medicine to facilitate Chinese medicine interaction research.

In our previous research, we proposed a literature analysis system for Chinese medicine [3]. In this paper, we further strengthen the system to visualize and predict medicine interactions related to Chinese medicine. We build an effective system to summarize

© Springer International Publishing AG 2017
C. Xing et al. (Eds.): ICSH 2016, LNCS 10219, pp. 155–165, 2017.
DOI: 10.1007/978-3-319-59858-1_15

and visualize the known interactions (for both Chinese and Western medicine) that are related to the known components of a focal Chinese medicine. In addition, we prediction possible but unknown interactions and connect such interactions to evidence in the literature to support physicians' work. We compare the performance of state-of-the-art interaction prediction algorithms in the paper.

2 Literature Review

2.1 Chinese Medicine Interactions

Traditional Chinese medicine is increasingly used with Western medicine in practice, especially to treat chronic diseases. An overview of traditional Chinese medicine can be found in [4]. In this study, we focus on the review of Chinese medicine interactions, which need to be taken care of in clinical practice.

There are studies on interactions of particular Chinese medicines. For instance, Guo et al. [5] analyzed the interactions of Rhizoma Chuanxiong. Wang et al. studied the interactions related to Liquorice [6]. Wen et al. studied the interaction between Danshensu and Rosuvastatin [7]. These studies collected fundamental evidence to direct the use of Chinese medicines.

Due to the integrative use of Chinese medicine and Western medicine, there is a need to study their interactions. Fugh-Berman discussed several key issues about interactions between herb medicine and Western medicine and gave a brief summary of interactions of several herb medicines [8, 9]. Later researchers continued to work on issues related to Chinese medicine interactions. Izzo studied clinical evidence of interactions between herb medicine and conventional medicine and created a detailed summarization table [10]. Izzo's work is valuable for healthcare professionals to prevent known interactions or adverse events of Chinese medicines. Long et al. discussed some aspects of interactions between Chinese medicine and Western medicine, such as characteristics, pharmacokinetics, and pharmacodynamics [11].

From a predictive analytics perspective, it is also possible to predict interactions between Chinese medicine and Western medicine to direct clinical experiments. However, there are limited studies on this problem. A fundamental work was conducted by Chan et al. [12], which proposed to extract constituent phytochemicals from traditional Chinese medicine and then use protein targets of extracted phytochemicals and some enzymes that play an important role in the metabolic procedure of drugs to predict potential herb-drug interactions. This method is based on the known mechanisms of specific enzymes for prediction, which limits its generalizability.

In general, the studies that provide a comprehensive understanding of interactions of Chinese medicines are still insufficient. A framework for discovering and predicting the interactions between Chinese medicines needs to be established.

2.2 Interaction Prediction in Western Medicine

As compared with Chinese medicines, research on the interactions among Western medicines is much more abundant. Those studies fall into two directions. The first direction is the classic biological approach, which examines interactions based on biological experiments [11–14]. Obach summarized recent advances and challenges of the biological approach [2]. However, conducting biological studies is costly. So, the second direction, using computational methods to predict potential interactions (and direct biological studies), is important in drug development.

One major stream of interaction prediction methods is the similarity-based approaches. Similarities between medicines can be calculated based on various information, such as compound structure, mechanism, and target. Zhang et al. [15] proposed an approach to predict drug-drug interactions based on side effect information. They constructed a similarity network of medicines first based on the compound structure and label/off-label side effects. Then, interactions can spread to the whole network from known interactions. Vilar et al. [16] proposed a matrix modeling approach that is applicable for large-scale interaction prediction. A potential medicine interaction matrix was derived by multiplying a standard interaction matrix and drug similarity matrix. Celebi et al. [17] proposed a link-prediction method to predict drug-drug interactions. They applied the Rooted PageRank algorithm for link prediction and compared it with several traditional methods such as distance graph, common neighbors, and Adamic/Adar. The similarity measures can also be used in machine learning algorithms to predict interactions [18, 19]. For example, Fokoue et al. [19] proposed to construct a link-link medicine similarity network and then apply Logistic Regression to predict drug-drug interactions. They combined several similarity measures and defined a new feature on the similarity of medicine links.

One challenge in extending studies on Western medicine to Chinese medicine is that a Chinese medicine usually contains several compounds; thus its interaction would be more complicated.

3   Medicine Interaction Analysis System

3.1   System Architecture

In our previous research, we developed MedC [3], a search system that indices Chinese medicine literature published in China and provides summarization/visualization. In this paper, we build on this previous effort and focus on presenting the interactions among Chinese medicines and connecting the interactions to clinical evidence in the literature.

The interaction analysis module is an important part of MedC. Figure 1 presents the interaction prediction procedure. First, we collect Chinese medicines and their component data. MedC focuses on the Chinese medicines recognized by the Hong Kong government[1] for analysis. In the prototype, a portion of the compound data is collected from the Shanghai Institute of Organic Chemistry's database[2] and temporarily used for the prototype demo.

---

[1] https://goo.gl/1WwfR7.

[2] http://www.organchem.csdb.cn/scdb/main/tcm_introduce.asp.

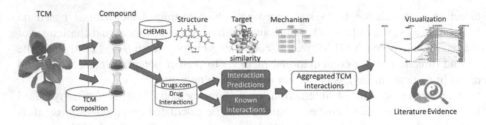

Fig. 1. System architecture of the medicine interaction analysis system

Second, after converting Chinese medicine to compounds, we collect interaction data of the compounds from drugs.com, which are from Western medicine research. Drugs.com provides three levels of interaction severity: major, moderate, and minor[3]. Major means that the interaction is highly clinically significant and the risk of the interaction outweighs the benefit; moderate means that doctors should avoid combining the two medicines; minor means that the interaction is minimally significant.

Third, we locate the compounds' characteristics in a Western medicine database, specifically, ChEMBL[4], a famous chemical database created/maintained by the European Bioinformatics Institute (EBI). From ChEMBL, we get a medicine's chemical property, mechanism, and targets. Based on characteristics of the components, we can identify similar medicines. Based on the known interactions and the similarities of compounds, possible interactions between components are predicted.

Finally, the system displays the path from Chinese medicines to compounds to the interacting compounds and Chinese medicines. The inferred Chinese medicines are then connected to clinical evidence in literature through the classic literature search function of MedC to help the users judge the validity of the predictions.

3.2   System Functionality

Basic functions of the MedC system were introduced in our previous paper [3]. In this paper, we focus on the interaction analysis module. To illustrate the functionalities of this system, imagine that a user aims to find interaction information for E-gelatin (阿胶), a widely used traditional Chinese medicine. Figure 2 shows the results web page after searching E-gelatin. On top of the literature containing E-gelatin, there is a brief introduction of the searched Chinese medicines, including Chinese name, English name, Latin name, catalog, brief description, function, and target. Below that is the interaction tree visualization map, which consists of four parts: the searched medicine, its known compounds, the Western medicine interacting with the compounds, and the related interacting Chinese medicine. There may exist multiple compounds that interact with the same set of medicines. To save space, the visualization combines such medicines in one interface and creates a network structure. If the mouse is put on the lines between the four parts, the entire interaction path will be highlighted to help users read the

---

3 https://www.drugs.com/drug_interactions.html.
4 https://www.ebi.ac.uk/chembl.

relationships. The interface also omits the links that do not link to any medicines for the sake of simplicity. The visualization is developed using JavaScript library d3[5]. The interaction tree is developed based on the parallel coordinates model[6].

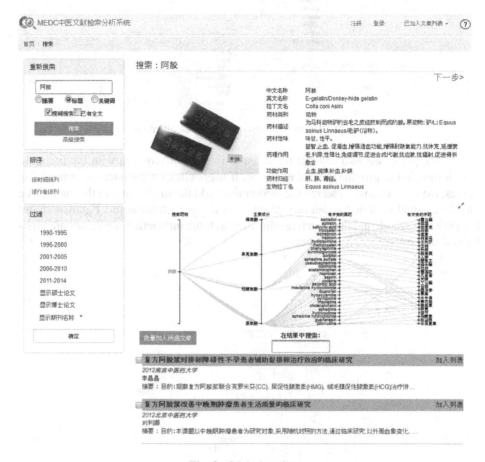

Fig. 2. Main interface

In addition to the aggregated view, there is an extended view of the interaction tree. As shown in Fig. 3, this view presents a detailed picture of Chinese medicine interactions, which does not merge compounds, and provides a full tree structure of different medicines.

---

[5] https.//d3js.org/.

[6] https://en.wikipedia.org/wiki/Parallel_coordinates.

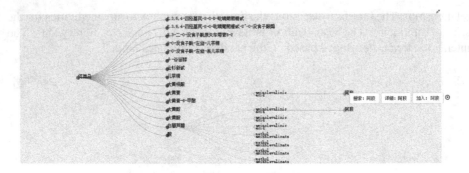

Fig. 3. The entire interaction tree visualization

On this page, we also connect the inferred interactions system with the literature search function to provide clinical evidence. If users click on the interacting medicine names, they can choose to search the medicine or add the medicine into the query. The interface can also show the detailed information about each medicine. Figure 4 shows the enriched search and the search results, in which the interacting medicines are highlighted to show the searched papers.

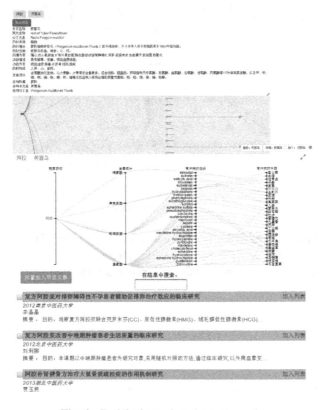

Fig. 4. Enriched search and search results

3.3   Medicine Interaction Prediction

The core function of our system is to analyze and predict Chinese medicine interactions. One challenge in Chinese medicine interaction is that a Chinese medicine usually contains several compounds and interacts with multiple medicines.

Suppose the component set of Chinese medicine x is denoted as

$$C_x = \{c_{xi}\}, c_{xi} = 1 \ if \ x \ contains \ i,$$

where x is a Chinese medicine and i is the compounds. Suppose we know drug interaction $D = \{d_{ij}\}$, where i, j are two compounds and $d_{ij} = 1, 2, 3$ is the interaction intensity. Then the overall interaction of two Chinese medicines x and y can be represented as $(C_x)D(C_y^T)$, where $()$ is the normalization operation.

Hence, predicting interaction between two Chinese medicines x, y can be transformed to predicting interactions between their components C_x, C_y. Thus, the fundamental problem for medicine interaction prediction is still to predict interactions between compounds. In this study, we adopt two similarity-based algorithms to predict interactions. If two compounds are similar, they may have similar interactions with other medicines. After interactions between compounds are predicted, interactions between Chinese medicine scan also be derived.

3.3.1   Compound Similarity

The similarity-based approach in this study takes a compound structure, target, and mechanism to calculate similarity. The structure similarity of compounds is calculated by the fingerprint method [4, 5], where the fingerprint is a binary vector with all information about the compound, such as the number of atoms and the number of bonds. Four fingerprints are used: FCPF4, ECPF4, topological, and MACCS. After fingerprints are computed, the Jaccard coefficient[7] is used to compute similarities between compounds as

$$S_{AB} = \frac{|A \cap B|}{|A| + |B| - |A \cap B|},$$

where A and B are two fingerprints.

In addition to structure similarities, we also calculate target similarity and mechanism similarity. The medicine's target in the body and mechanism of action are both collected from drugs.com as vectors. Thus, the Jaccard coefficient is also used to compute their similarities.

---

[7] Other measurements such as Dice coefficient or Cosine coefficient can also be used. But the Jaccard coefficient is the most widely used measurement for calculating structure similarity.

3.3.2   Interaction Prediction

In this study, we adopt two interaction prediction algorithms, the Logistic Regression method, and the matrix modeling approach.

The Logistic Regression method [6] creates a link-link similarity feature derived from medicine similarity. It transforms drug-drug similarity to interaction-interaction similarity. Then, a Logistic Regression model is trained to predict potential interactions. The link-link similarity is calculated as

$$SIM((a1, a2), (b1, b2)) = average\left(S_{a_1 b_1}, S_{a_2 b_2}\right),$$

where $(a1, a2)$ and $(b1, b2)$ are two links among medicines, and S_{a1b1} (S_{a2b2}) is the similarity between a_1 and b_1 $(a_2$ and $b_2)$. Let D be the set of a known drug-drug interaction. The method defines $F(d_1, d_2)$ upon two drugs d_1 and d_2 as their most similar pair in D

$$F\left(d_1, d_2\right) = max\left\{ SIM\left(\left(d_1, d_2\right), (x, y)\right) \middle| (x, y) \in D - \left\{\left(d_1, d_2\right)\right\} \right\}.$$

Based on the new link-link feature, Logistic Regression is used to predict interactions.

The matrix modeling approach [7] constructs one similarity matrix S_k for each similarity measure and leverages the known interaction matrix D to predict potential interactions. In drug similarity matrix S_k, the diagonal elements are set to 0. By multiplying D and S_k, we have $M_k = DS_k$. The predicted interaction M is set as

$$M = max\_cell(M_k : M_k^T),$$

where $max\_cell(M_k : M_k^T)$ retains higher value in each cell of matrices M_k and M_k^T. Finally, the value of M can be used as the confidence level to sort and predict interactions. Because we have six types of similarity, the six types of predictions can generate a combined score of potential interactions.

4   Interaction Prediction Algorithm Comparison

4.1   Dataset

Our Chinese medicine database contains 352 Chinese medicines extracted from the literature. They are composed of 1,366 compounds, i.e., Western medicines. We collect these medicines' characteristics from ChEMBL. From drugs.com we collect the interactions of the 4,696 compounds. We identify 128,535 interactions among the 1,366 compounds. On average, there are 94 interactions per drug. The largest number of interactions is 837. Figure 5 shows the degree distribution of the drugs in the drug interaction relationships.

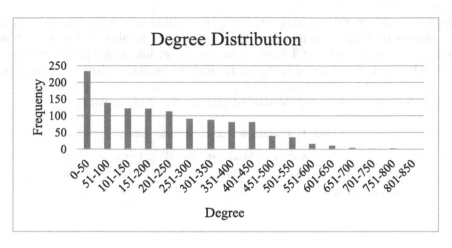

Fig. 5. Degree distribution

4.2 Experiment Framework

In our experiment, we conduct 10-fold cross validation to evaluate the performance of the two algorithms. In 10-fold cross validation, known interaction D is divided into 10 subsets. In each round, one subset is chosen as the validation set and the other 9 subsets are used for training. After prediction, the performance is measured by comparing the prediction results with the validation set. The overall performance is calculated by integrating all ten results.

In this study, we use the widely used accuracy, precision, recall, and F-score as evaluation metrics to measure the quality of prediction. Accuracy is the correctly predicted interactions in all interactions. Precision is the proportion of correctly predicted interactions in all predicted interactions. Recall is the proportion of correctly predicted items in all known interactions. F-score combines precision and recall as

$$F = 2 \cdot \frac{P \cdot R}{P + R}.$$

Moreover, we use the area under the receiver operating characteristic curve (AUROC) to report the overall performance of different predictions.

4.3 Result

Table 1 shows the result of the two medicines prediction algorithms. Obviously, the overall performance of Matrix Modeling is better than Logistic Regression, which can be considered in further system implementation. Compared with Matrix Modeling, all measurements of Logistic Regression are worse, especially for precision, recall, and F-score. That means Matrix Modeling has a better performance on finding True Positive examples, i.e. correct potential interactions. The reason for the worse performance of Logistic Regression may be the unbalance positive and negative instances in the training set. There are much more non-interaction pairs in the training set than interactions. We have reduced the number of non-interaction pairs in training set to about 3 times of the number of interaction pairs and implemented the method introduced in [6], but the improvement is limited. If we continue to reduce the number of non-interaction pairs, the accuracy of prediction decreased rapidly. So how to handle the unbalanced data remains a big problem.

Table 1. Interaction Prediction Performance

	Accuracy	Precision	Recall	F-score	AUROC
Logistic regression	0.818	0.330	0.367	0.348	0.686
Matrix modeling	0.866	0.497	0.545	0.520	0.715

5   Conclusion

In this paper, we constructed a Chinese medicine analysis and prediction framework based on the existing MedC literature analysis system. We conduct Chinese medicine interaction analysis on the interactions of compounds of Chinese medicine. We build an effective system to summarize and visualize the interactions that are related to Chinese medicines. In addition, we connect such interactions to evidence in the literature to support physicians' work. We also implemented and compared two state-of-the-art interaction prediction algorithms in the paper.

There is room to further improve the system. First, we will study how to convert predicted interactions of components to predicting the interactions with Chinese medicines. Second, due to the limitation of our data source, we only have a subset of the components of Chinese medicine. We will improve the database coverage in future. Third, we will conduct further study and propose new interaction prediction algorithms.

Acknowledgements. The research is partially supported by GuangDong Science and Technology Project 2014A020221090 and the City University of Hong Kong Shenzhen Research Institute.

References

1. Dobos, G., Tao, I.: The model of western integrative medicine: the role of Chinese medicine. Chin. J. Integr. Med. **17**(1), 11–20 (2011)
2. Obach, R.S.: Predicting drug-drug interactions from in vitro drug metabolism data: challenges and recent advances. Curr. Opin. Drug Discov. Dev. **12**(1), 81–89 (2009)
3. Li, X., Tong, Yu., Wang, W.: MedC: a literature analysis system for Chinese medicine research. In: Zheng, X., Zeng, D.D., Chen, H., Leischow, S.J. (eds.) ICSH 2015. LNCS, vol. 9545, pp. 311–320. Springer, Cham (2016). doi:10.1007/978-3-319-29175-8_29
4. Lao, L., Xu, L., Xu, S.: Traditional Chinese medicine. In: Längler, A., Mansky, P.J., Seifert, G. (eds.) Integrative Pediatric Oncology, pp. 125–135. Springer, Heidelberg (2012)

5. Guo, M., Su, X., Kong, L., Li, X., Zou, H.: Characterization of interaction property of multicomponents in Chinese herb with protein by microdialysis combined with HPLC. Anal. Chim. Acta **556**(1), 183–188 (2006)
6. Wang, X., Zhang, H., Chen, L., Shan, L., Fan, G., Gao, X.: Liquorice, a unique 'guide drug' of traditional Chinese medicine: a review of its role in drug interactions. J. Ethnopharmacol. **150**(3), 781–790 (2013)
7. Wen, J., Wei, X., Cheng, X.: OATP1B1 in drug-drug interactions between traditional Chinese medicine Danshensu and Rosuvastatin. Yao Xue Xue Bao **51**(1), 75–79 (2016)
8. Fugh-Berman, A., Ernst, E.: Herb ± drug interactions: review and assessment of report reliability. Br. J. Clin. Pharmacol. **52**, 587–595 (2001)
9. Fugh-Berman, A.: Herb-drug interactions. Lancet **355**, 134–138 (2000)
10. Izzo, A.A.: Interactions between herbs and conventional drugs: overview of the clinical data. Med. Princ. Pract. **21**(5), 404–428 (2012)
11. Long, X., Li, H., Zhan, Y.-F.: Exploration on interaction of Chinese and Western drugs. Chin. J. Integr. Tradit. West. Med. **29**(5), 457–460 (2009)
12. Chan, E., Tan, M., Xin, J., Sudarsanam, S., Johnson, D.E.: Interactions between traditional Chinese medicines and Western therapeutics. Curr. Opin. Drug Discov. Dev. **13**(1), 50–65 (2010)
13. Obach, R.S., Walsky, R.L., Venkatakrishnan, K.: Mechanism-based inactivation of human cytochrome P450 enzymes and the prediction of drug-drug interactions. Drug Metab. Dispos. **35**(2), 246–255 (2007)
14. Bjornsson, T.D., Callaghan, J.T., Einolf, H.J., Fischer, V.: The conduct of in vitro and in vivo drug-drug interaction studies: a PhRMA perspective. J. Clin. Pharmacol. **43**(5), 443–469 (2003)
15. Zhang, P., Wang, F., Hu, J., Sorrentino, R.: Label propagation prediction of drug-drug interactions based on clinical side effects. Sci. Rep. **5**, 12339 (2015)
16. Vilar, S., Uriarte, E., Santana, L., Lorberbaum, T.: Similarity-based modeling in large-scale prediction of drug-drug interactions. Nat. Protoc. **9**(9), 2147–2163 (2014)
17. Celebi, R., Mostafapour, V., Yasar, E., Gumus, O., Dikenelli, O.: Prediction of drug-drug interactions using pharmacological similarities of drugs. In: Proceedings of the International Workshop Database and Expert Systems Applications (DEXA), pp. 14–17 (2016)
18. Cheng, F., Zhao, Z.: Machine learning-based prediction of drug-drug interactions by integrating drug phenotypic, therapeutic, chemical, and genomic properties. J. Am. Med. Inform. Assoc. **21**(e2), e278–e286 (2014)
19. Fokoue, A., Hassanzadeh, O., Sadoghi, M., Zhang, P.: Predicting drug-drug interactions through similarity-based link prediction over web data. In: Proceedings of the 25th International Conference on Companion World Wide Web, pp. 3–6 (2016)

Classification of Cataract Fundus Image Based on Retinal Vascular Information

Yanyan Dong[1], Qing Wang[2], Qinyan Zhang[1], and Jijiang Yang[2(✉)]

[1] Automation School, Beijing University of Post
and Telecommunications, Beijing, China
dyy0506@bupt.edu.cn, zh_qinyan@l63.com
[2] Research Institute of Information Technology, Tsinghua University,
Beijing 100084, China
qing.wang@tsinghua.edu.cn, yangjijiang@tsingha.edu.cn

Abstract. Cataract is a dulling or clouding of the lens inside the eye. Which is one of the most common diseases that might cause blindness. Considering the damage impact of cataract, we propose to use retinal vascular information for automatic cataract detection, which based on the classification of retinal image. This method focus on the preprocessing step of retinal image. Firstly, we use the maximum entropy method to enhance the contract level of fundus image. Next, in order to collect vessel information based on the Kirsh template of multi-layer filter is used. Last, adaptive weighted median filter has proposed to reduce the noise of the image. Then, according to the retinal blood vessel image, we extracted wavelet features, texture features for cataract classification. For each set of features, SVMs (support vector machines) is used for cataract classification. Finally, cataract image classified into normal, slight, medium or severe four-class. Through comparing the result of classification, three of four classes obtains the better accuracy than former. At the same time, the time that spend on feature extract is greatly reduced. The result demonstrate that our research on classification system is effective and has practical value.

Keywords: Retinal image preprocessing · Cataract · Maximum entropy method · Kirsh template of multi-layer filter · Adaptive weighted median filter · Retinal blood vessel

1 Introduction

With the popularity of electronic devices in modern society, people have the growing demand on using eye. So eye protection becomes increasingly important in the daily.

Cataracts, diabetic retinopathy, conjunctivitis, glaucoma and other eye disease is the most common eye disease, they may even cause blindness in humans [1]. Cataract is the world's first cause of blindness. In our country there are 5 million cataract patients, nearly 1 million new patients each year. Prevention and treatment of cataracts is a challenge we have to face [1].

The original version of this chapter was revised: The third and fourth authors' affiliations were corrected. The erratum to this chapter is available at https://doi.org/10.1007/978-3-319-59858-1_24

© Springer International Publishing AG 2017
C. Xing et al. (Eds.): ICSH 2016, LNCS 10219, pp. 166–173, 2017.
DOI: 10.1007/978-3-319-59858-1_16

The traditional cataract treatment, the patient's eye is observed by an experience ophthalmologist directly by dialysis lamp, and computer classifiers have been proposed later to improve the accuracy and efficiency of diagnosis [2]. However, due to the number of cases and the algorithm performance, through the traditional machine learning methods, it has been difficult to obtain more excellent classification results, so we turn to the pre-processing and feature extraction of fundus images, do something different work, and have received better results in some areas. Figure 1 shows the cataract fundus images in different grading.

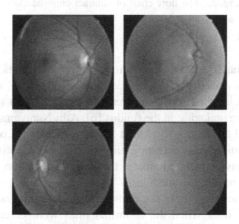

Fig. 1. The image of each grading. (a) normal; (b) slight; (c) medium; (d) severe

Only observe the degree of chaos on the fundus image, it is difficult to determine the degree of illness by the naked eye accurately, Except severe degree, others have neurovascular information.

In this paper we propose a comprehension pre-processing method. Figure 2 shows the flow chart of complete classification identification process. It mainly contains three parts, which are fundus image preprocessing, feature extraction, and automatic cataract classification and grading [3, 4]. Our research focuses on the image preprocessing. For feature extraction step, we use blood vessel wavelet feature and texture feature.

After feature extraction, SVM (support vector machine) and Staking are used for cataract classification [5]. The result in this paper proved that fundus image after a comprehensive preprocessing method to extract retinal blood vessels can get better classification effect and practical value.

The paper is organized accordingly: Sect. 2 describes related work. Section 3 gives out the implementation, and conclusion respectively.

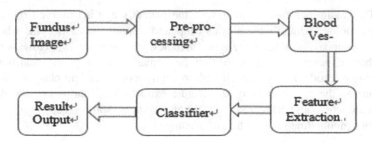

Fig. 2. The flow chart of cataract classification

2   Related Work

Research on fundus images analysis has been made for years. Joes Staal et al. extracted fundus blood vessels based on the characteristics of blood vessel skeleton [7]. Sidalingaswamy et al. applied repeated threshold segmentation method based on its luminance to search the optic disc in the fundus [6]. Athi Narayanan propose functional multilayer filter based on matrix to extract the fundus images of blood vessels [8]. AliShaik tried to impulse noise detection and filtering by adaptive weighted median filter [9]. His research effectively eliminates the noise distribution, and provides a new way for future image processing methods.

Michael applied the classifier to the retina. The retinal images were classified into normal and abnormal ones. Then the abnormal ones were given to the doctor, this greatly improve doctors' efficiency. Yang classified the diabetic retinal images into normal, mild, medium and severe ones. Zeng had put forword ensemble learning algorithm to improve the accuracy of classification [5]. He made a perfect job. Fan tried to use PCA (principal component analysis) to reduce the dimension of the image, but also get a good performance [10].

However, we find that it is more and more difficult to use the algorithm classifier to obtain other advantages. At the same time, there is little work focusing on preprocessing of fundus image. So we decide to take action about preprocessing and hope to get a better result.

3   Fundus Image Pre-processing

3.1   Maximum Entropy Contrast

Image enhancement is a key step in the pre-process of fundus image. In the past, we used the histogram equalization to enhance quality of image, but it will lose a lot of image information, and don't highlight the blood vessels of the fundus image information. On the basis of the principle of maximum entropy, the optimal classification threshold of gray level of the image is calculated by using the iterative algorithm, and then the local gray level transformation is performed by the transform function. Take the gray level of the images edge, by finding the best separation point, then get the threshold value on both sides and improve function of nonlinear stretching in the spatial domain. In order to highlight the target brightness contrast of the image.

$$H(X) = \sum_{i=1}^{k} p(x = x_i) \log \frac{1}{p(x = x_i)} \tag{1}$$

$$H(x) = -\sum p(x) \log \frac{1}{p(x)} \tag{2}$$

$$0 \le H(X) \le \log|X| \tag{3}$$

$$H_{max}(T) = -\sum_{x=x_{min}}^{T} U(x) \cdot P_a(x \cdot \log(U_a(x) \cdot P_a(x))$$
$$-\sum_{x=T+1}^{x_{min}} U_b(x) \cdot P_b(x) \cdot \log(U_b(x) \cdot P_b(x)) \tag{4}$$

After the maximum entropy contrast enhancement, the changes of the fundus images are as follows Fig. 3.

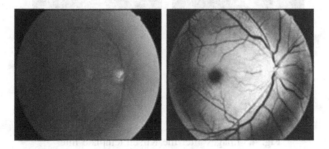

Fig. 3. (a) Original image and (b) image after maximum entropy contrast

3.2 Kirsch Template Filter

After contrast enhancement, the fundus blood vessel information greatly improved, so we propose to take convolution for each pixel on the image, derivative of the 8 template represents the 8 directions, in order to make the large response to 8 specific edge direction on the image with Kirsch's 8 template operator, the edge of the image is max output operation.

$$H1 = \frac{1}{15} \begin{vmatrix} 5 & -3 & -3 \\ 5 & 0 & -3 \\ 5 & -3 & -3 \end{vmatrix} \quad H2 = \frac{1}{15} \begin{vmatrix} -3 & -3 & 5 \\ -3 & 0 & 5 \\ -3 & -3 & 5 \end{vmatrix} \quad H3 = \frac{1}{15} \begin{vmatrix} -3 & -3 & -3 \\ 5 & 0 & -3 \\ 5 & 5 & -3 \end{vmatrix}$$

$$H4 = \frac{1}{15} \begin{vmatrix} -3 & 5 & 5 \\ -3 & 0 & 5 \\ 5 & 5 & -3 \end{vmatrix} \quad H5 = \frac{1}{15} \begin{vmatrix} -3 & -3 & -3 \\ -3 & 0 & -3 \\ 5 & 5 & 5 \end{vmatrix} \quad H6 = \frac{1}{15} \begin{vmatrix} 5 & 5 & 5 \\ -3 & 0 & -3 \\ -3 & -3 & -3 \end{vmatrix}$$

$$H7 = \frac{1}{15} \begin{vmatrix} -3 & -3 & -3 \\ -3 & 0 & 5 \\ -3 & 5 & 5 \end{vmatrix} \quad H8 = \frac{1}{15} \begin{vmatrix} 5 & 5 & -3 \\ 5 & 0 & -3 \\ -3 & -3 & -3 \end{vmatrix}$$

After filtering the template of these eight kinds of operators, we hope to use the Laplace operator which is independent on the edge direction, so that it strengthens the edge of the fundus blood vessel. The formula is as follows

$$\nabla^2 f(x,y) = \frac{\partial^2 f(x,y)}{\partial x^2} + \frac{\partial^2 f(x,y)}{\partial y^2} \tag{5}$$

$$G[i,j] = |f[i+1,j] + f[i-1,j] + f[i,j+1] + f[i,j-1] - 4f[i,j]| \tag{6}$$

Laplace operator is sensitive to noise, and the noise is enhanced, but the blood vessels in the fundus image can be extracted as much as possible, which provides the possibility for the following research. After the Kirsch template filter, the changes of the fundus images are as follows Fig. 4.

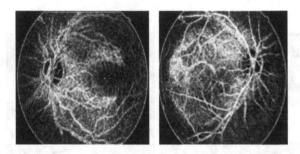

Fig. 4. Images after the Kirsch template filter

3.3   Adaptive Weighted Median Filter

We use the adaptive weighted median filter to eliminate the noise of the image, at the same time protect the edge of the blood vessel as possible. Firstly, according to the number of noise points in the window, determine the window size of filter adaptively; next, take the weighted median filter algorithm adaptively to determine the weight of each pixel in the filter window.

When the noise points of the image are determined, the 3 * 3 window is used to slide on the image, and the gray value of the window center pixel (x, y) is seen as p(x, y). Threshold is defined as d:

$$\frac{1}{3}\sqrt{\sum_{i=1}^{i}\sum_{j=1}^{j}\left|f(i+k,j+r) - \frac{1}{9}\sum_{i=1}^{i}\sum_{j=1}^{j}f(i+k,j+r)\right|} \tag{7}$$

Standard median filtering algorithm to remove the noise is affected by the size of the filter window. That the filter window is small can better protect the image details, There is a great correlation in a neighborhood of the central pixel point. In order to describe the filtering window of a pixel (I + k, j + r) gray value is seen as f (I + k, j + r), the degree of similarity of the sampling window center pixel gray value is (F, I, J). After computational similarity, the filtering window center pixel (I, J) is weighted median filter, and the corresponding gray value is obtained.

$$g(i,j) = Weighted\_Med \left\{ \begin{array}{c} f(i=n,j=n), f(i=n,j=n+1), \\ \cdot \\ \cdots, f(i,j) \cdots, f(i+n,j+n) \end{array} \right\} \quad (8)$$

The noise of the fundus image has obviously reduced after filtering. The changes of each category fundus images are as follows Fig. 5.

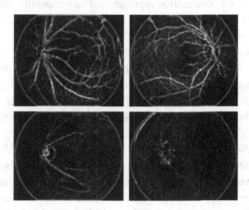

Fig. 5. Each category of image after adaptive weighted median filter

4   Classification and Accuracy

After the step of preprocessing, we use Matlab to carry out the wavelet and texture feature extraction. Then SVM and the Staking algorithm is used to classify the wavelet and texture features of test set.

SVM (support vector machines) are a very popular learning algorithm, which can be used for classification and regression, the principle is mapping the low dimensional input space into higher dimension feature, then we use the kernel function which is determined through test set, to obtain the relaxation coefficient and the penalty coefficient. Last, we use test data to test accuracy of the classification.

Staking algorithm is a kind of famous integrated learning method. It begins with an initial training set build primary study, generating a new data set for training secondary learning period. This tries also to get a good result.

Table 1. Divided into four-class by using SVM

Features	Normal (%)	Slight (%)	Medium (%)	Severe (%)	Overall mean
Wavelet	94.91	75.13	90.47	0	81.81
Texture	91.54	70	76.19	62.5	80.33

Table 2. Divided into four-class by using staking algorithm

Normal (%)	Slight (%)	Medium (%)	Severe (%)	Overall mean (%)
94.91	77.27	80.95	50.2	84

5 The Result Analysis

We collected 445 fundus images, the normal is 199, the slight is 148, the medium is 71 and the severe is 27. These fundus images are classified by the professional doctor working in the department of ophthalmology, 70% randomly selected samples from the data used for training the classification algorithm. The remaining 30% is used to test the accuracy of classifiers. After repeated training and testing for 50 times, we obtained the overall performance of the classification.

Tables 1 and 2 show the classification results of four-class by using SVMs and Staking respectively. And in these two tables we know that the highest overall mean value is 94.91%, which are results of wavelet features, 3.37% higher than the result texture feature. The overall mean of Staking is 84%, 2.19% higher than the correct rate of wavelet features which value is 84.34%, and 3.67% higher than texture feature. Comparing with Zeng's research, which the correct rate of wavelet features and texture feature is 80.3%, 79.54% respectively. Our research also have 1.51%, 0.79% superior than his. About the best accuracy rate of fundus classification, his Staking accuracy is 82.57%, we also have slight greater performance. Through the above discussion we know the best accuracy rate of fundus classification is 84%. It has slight improve in accuracy compare with previous work [7]. Adaptive weighted median filter. It is just 45 s that we can get a pre-processed fundus image. This step saves at least 80% of preprocess time than previous. The study has the extremely vital significance for practical research.

6 Conclusion

Kirsch Template Filter and adaptive weighted median filter is proposed to preprocess of fundus image to extract vascular information. It has great progress in consume time of preprocess. Though it not has lot superior accurate rate than previous, but it is the first try in our research. In the actual diagnosis of cataract, there is little possibility to treat a severe cataract patients to recovery, so the doctor emphasis focuses on the slight and medium performance. In this research, we have a good performance in core level.

In the future, we will continue our research with emphasis on extracting the feature of blood vessel by better segmentation algorithm. Furthermore, deep learning will be also used to get better accuracy.

Acknowledgment. This research is supported by following grants: China National Key Research and Development Program with No. 2013BAH19F01.

References

1. http://www.iapb.org/vision-2020
2. Staal, J., Abramoff, M.D., et al.: Ridge based vessel segmentation in color images of the retina. IEEE Trans. Med. Image **23**(4), 501–509 (2004)
3. Yang, M., Yang, J., Zhang, Q., Niu, Y., Li, J.: Classification of retinal image for automatic cataract detection. In: 2013 IEEE 15th International Conference on e-Health Networking, Application & Service (Health com), 9 October, pp. 674–679 (2013)
4. Guo, L., Yang, J., Peng, L., Li, J.: A computer-aided healthcare system for cataract classification and grading based on fundus image analysis. Comput. Ind. **69**, 72–78 (2015)
5. Zeng, Y.: Classification of cataract fundus images based on ensemble learning algorithm
6. Siddalingaswamy, P.C., Prabhu, G.K.: Automated detection of anatomical structures in retinal images. In: International Conference, vol. 3, pp. 164–168 (2007)
7. Orlandoa, J.I., del Fresnoac, M.: Review pre-processing feature extraction technical for retinal blood vessel segmentation in fundus image (2014)
8. Athinarayanan, S., Srinath, M.V.: Multi class cervical cancer classification in pap smear images using hybrid texture feature and fuzzy logical based SVM. Int. J. Recent Sci. Res. **7**(2), 8831–8837 (2016)
9. Xiuqin, D., Yong, X., Hong, P.: Effective adaptive weighted median filter algorithm. Comput. Eng. Appl. **45**(35), 185–187 (2009)
10. Weiming, F.: Principal component analysis based cataract grading and classification. In: 2015 IEEE 17th International Conference on e-Health Networking, Application & Service (Health com), 9 October, pp. 674–679 (2015)

Medical Data Machine Translation Evaluation Based on Dependency N-Grams

Ying Qin[✉] and Ye Liang

Beijing Foreign Studies University, Beijing 100089, China
{qinying,liangye}@bfsu.edu.cn

Abstract. Machine Translation is increasingly applied to medical cross-lingual data processing. In order to evaluate the quality of machine translation, automatic evaluation approaches like BLEU and NIST, most of which are n-gram based metrics, are widely used besides costly human evaluation. Current evaluation approaches merely make surface linguistic comparisons between the candidate and reference translations. Furthermore the domain features such medical terms, dependent and cohesive relations in and among sentences in medical documents should be taken into account when evaluating translations. However severe noises are imported into the procedure when faulty machine translations are parsed using the current syntactic parsers. Therefore using the noisy parsing results to compare with references affects the improvement of evaluation even though the deep processing is incorporated. To lessen noises as well as grasp the main meaning of a sentence, the paper proposes to extract the dependency n-grams only based on dependency parsing of reference translations. Dependency n-grams are stemmed and extended according to linguistic rules and then viewed as the key points for quality evaluation. The score of candidate translation is computed according to the count of dependency n-grams loose matching. Also the penalty of short translation and the clip count of the highest frequency of dependency n-grams are incorporated in the final score of the candidate. Experiments on our translation datasets show the evaluation based on dependency n-grams significantly outperforms the metric of BLEU and NSIT. This approach is also significantly better than the related research which employs dependency relation parsing in evaluation.

Keywords: Medical data · Machine Translation Quality Evaluation · Dependency relation parsing · Dependency n-grams

1   Introduction

Recently multilingual medical resources and information have raised much interest in smart health community. New technology like Machine Translation (MT) has been applied to cross-lingual medical information processing. The demand of high quality medical translative documents is the main driving force of study in automatic evaluation approach. Reference-based evaluation metrics such as BLEU [7] and NIST [3], which are the *de facto* metrics in Workshop of Machine

© Springer International Publishing AG 2017
C. Xing et al. (Eds.): ICSH 2016, LNCS 10219, pp. 174–181, 2017.
DOI: 10.1007/978-3-319-59858-1_17

Translation (WMT), compare machine translations with the human translations: the more similar the better quality they will have. However the varieties of acceptable translations make the superficial comparison unable to capture the semantic similarities between candidate translation and references. Moreover many meaningless n-grams such as *are one of the, to a* are created [8] but medical terms which generally play more important roles than these nonsense word sequences. Therefore some researchers try deeper level analysis on translations such as LFG [6], syntactic, constitute parsing and dependency relation [5,9]. But the outcomes of evaluation are not satisfying.

To be noticed that most machine translations are not perfect translations. When they are parsed by the current syntactic parsers a lot of severe noises are introduced, which cause the comparison unfeasible. The research on lexis in translations of drug package inserts [10] shows that the main cohesive types and subcategories in English and Chinese translations have the same distributions. The result confirms that the dependency and cohesion relation will help to explore the deeper similarities in quality evaluation.

In the paper we proposed translation quality evaluation algorithm based on core semantic n-grams extracted from dependency parsing of reference translations, hereinafter referred as dependency n-grams. Some open syntactic n-grams resources like Google n-grams have been successfully used to the natural language processing tasks [8]. Our experiments on the dependency n-grams evaluation approach show that the approach not only outperforms the traditional n-gram based algorithm BLEU and NIST but also has a higher efficiency.

In the section follows we briefly review the BLEU and NIST metric. In Sect. 3 we discuss the ways of dependency n-grams extraction and how to make use of dependency n-grams in translation quality evaluation. Experiments on 1797 sentences (from Chinese into English) are presented in Sect. 4. We also compare the performance with a related research on dependency parsing.

2   Review of N-grams Based Evaluation

2.1   BLEU

By exhaustedly enumerating the word sequences in references and searching in the candidate translations, BLEU algorithm accumulates the common n-grams between the candidate and references. The BLEU score of candidate translation is given in Eq. 1 [7].

$$S\_BLEU = BP \times exp \sum_{n=1}^{N} w_n log P_n,$$ (1)

where

$$P_n = \frac{\sum_{C \in Candi} \sum_{ngram \in C} Count_{clip}(ngram)}{\sum_{C \in Candi} \sum_{ngram' \in C'} Count(ngram')}$$

$$BP = \begin{cases} 1, & if\ |c| \geq |r| \\ e^{(1-|r|/|c|)}, & if\ |c| < |r| \end{cases}$$

w_n is a weighting factor usually set as $1/N$, where N is the longest possible n-gram considered by the matching method. N is usually set to 4 to avoid data sparseness issues resulting from longer n-grams. P_n is the n-gram precision at a given n and in essence represents the proportion of n-grams in the candidate translation that also appear in the reference translation. BP is a penalty factor for shorter segments. c and r are the length of the candidate segment and reference segment, respectively. Due to the sparsity of n-grams with large n and the geometric average of n-gram precisions, BLEU is not suitable for sentence-level evaluation. Several smoothing approaches have been proposed to alleviate this issue, such as the standard plus-one smoothing [4] and combinations of smoothing techniques [1].

2.2   NIST

NIST is an improvement on BLEU in that n-grams are weighted according to the value information. So the less frequent n-grams are weighted heavier than those which occur frequently. Additionally the geometry average is replaced by arithmetic average in the finally score to avoid 0.

The NIST metric weights n-grams that occur less frequently in references more heavily [3], as shown in Eq. 2.

$$S\_NIST = \sum_{n=1}^{N} \left\{ \sum_{\substack{w_1...w_n \\ co-occur}} Info(w_1 \ldots w_n) / \sum_{\substack{w_1...w_n \\ \text{in system}}} (1) \right\}$$

$$\times \ exp \left\{ \beta log_2 \left[min(\frac{L_{sys}}{\overline{L_{ref}}}, 1) \right] \right\}, \tag{2}$$

where

$$Info(w_1 \ldots w_n) = log(\frac{\text{\# of occur of } w_1 \ldots w_{n-1}}{\text{\# of occur of } w_1 \ldots w_n})$$

and $\overline{L_{ref}}$ is the average number of words in all references, L_{sys} is the number of words in the system translation, β is used as a weight for the penalty factor, and N is often set as 5.

The NIST metric focuses on non-popular n-grams in references and assumes that highly frequent n-grams, such as function words which tend to carry little meaning. However, this method consequently weakens the validity of medical terms that recur in multiple references.

To summarize, there will be a large number of meaningless n-grams in the above two n-grams based translation quality evaluation algorithms which can not reflect the real quality of translated medical data.

3   Dependency N-gram Based Evaluation

According to the theory of dependency grammar, the basic units in a sentence are dependent on each other by kinds of relations, forming the complete structure of the sentence. Generally the core of a sentence is verb. However the dependent relations is not decided by neighboring and order of words. A dependent relation consists of a head and its dependency. We use the famous Stanford University dependency parser CoreNLP[1] to parse the experimental data which provides as many as 50 dependent relations of English sentence. Here is an instance of dependency parsing, shown in Fig. 1.

  (1) Clinicians should be aware of potential nutritional and metabolic problems and their consequences.

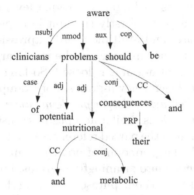

Fig. 1. Dependency relation parsing of sentence (1)

Some researchers have explored the dependent relations in machine translation evaluation. Liu et al. [5] extract the core word sequences of both candidate translation and reference, that is the bigram of head word of each dependent relation, and count the number of matching. For instance, in the above sentence parsed, the core word sequences they extracted are *aware clinicians, aware problems, aware should, aware be, problems of, problems potential....* The core word sequences is the reflection of related words in a sentence. To be noticed that the core word sequences are not as the same word order as in the translation. If there is no core word sequence matching, the advantage of dependency parsing will be lowered. Further researches on using dependent relations are implemented by [9]. They compare the dependent word sequence as well as dependent relations. Lexical Function Grammar (LFG) is also studied to extract the dependent trigrams denoted as (relation type, related word1, related word2). There are some improvements on evaluation but not significant.

We closely check the parsing result of machine translation and references and find there are too many errors in paring results, especially when parsing

---

[1] http://nlp.standford.edu:8080.

the machine translation. Although sentence (1) is the human translation, the parser output questionable dependency relations shown in Fig. 1. Therefore we speculate the advantage of dependency parsing is overwhelmed by parsing errors.

Actually lots of machine translations are faulty translations. We cannot assume all machine translations well-formed sentences. So the parsing of machine translation is not as useful as expected. On the other hand since the reference translations are well-formed sentences, we can extract the dependent n-grams, which contain the core semantic relations and keep the original order in references, then search in the candidate. In order to differ whether the word sequences are continuous or not, we use a special label ... to separate non-continuous words. For example, the dependency n-grams exacted from sentence (1) are as following.

clinicians...aware, aware...problems, aware of, potential problems, nutritional ... problems, problems ... consequences, ...

Most dependency n-grams are bigrams though, they are different with the traditional bigrams in four aspects. Firstly the unit in dependency n-grams is not only words but also phrases and Multiple Word Expressions (MWE). Therefore the actual length of dependency n-grams can be much larger than two. Secondly the continuity requirement of n-grams is loosed. So long distance matching can be captured by using the dependency n-grams. For example, dependency n-gram *aware...problems* can match *aware deeper problems, aware nutrition problem* and so on, which can cater to various similar acceptable translations. Thirdly dependency n-grams extracted from the parsed references usually carry the key meaning of a sentence avoiding the large amount of noisy n-grams. Lastly dependency n-grams can easily be extended into meaningful n-grams. For example, the preposition phrase *prep_of* can induce a noun phrase by moving the modifier to the front of the noun. Besides prepositional of structure, we also find several meaningful extension of some dependency n-grams according to linguistic rules as listed below.

- without or with conjunction in coordinate relation, e.g. *big and heavy -> big heavy*
- word order in coordinate relation, e.g. *malnutrition, obesity and cardiometabolic -> obesity, malnutrition and cardiometabolic*
- noun phrase with determiner, e.g. *a child -> child, the child*
- passive voice and active voice, e.g. *defeated -> was defeated*

In most circumstances the extensions are meaningful and helpful to capture more semantic similarity between candidate translation and references. The above analysis is summarized into the stages of dependency n-gram translation quality evaluation as:

- Parsing the reference translations
- Extracting dependency n-grams
- Dependency n-gram extension
- Dependency n-gram pattern
- Counting common dependency n-grams between candidate and references
- Calculating precision, recall and the final score

With regard to the length of candidate translation, we also add the penalty factor to the final score to lessen the effect of too short sentences. The penalty is defined same to BLEU. Considering all the factors, precision, recall and the final score are listed in the Eq. 3.

$$Pre = \frac{\sum\limits_{dngram \in Candidates} count_{clip}(word\ in\ dngram)}{\sum\limits_{word \in Candidates} count\ (word)}$$

$$Rec = \frac{\sum\limits_{dngram \in Candidates} count_{clip}(dngram)}{\sum\limits_{dngram' \in References} count_{clip}(dngram')}$$

$$Score_{dngram} = BP * \frac{2*Rec*Pre}{Rec + Pre} \tag{3}$$

4 Experiment

4.1 Datasets

Due to the rareness of bilingual medical corpus, we collect small scale of Chinese into English texts and use online machine translation system Google[2], Baidu[3] and Yeeyun[4] to translate Chinese medical document into English. The total experimental dataset contains 1797 sentences. Human raters are senior medical school students with good English. The human evaluation is scaled to 5 levels, the higher level representing the better quality. The inner consistence of human judgments on segment level is measured by the Cohen's Kappa coefficient [2], which is only fair: 0.227 on fluency and 0.172 on accuracy annotation.

4.2 Results and Analysis

The pipeline of dependency n-gram based translation quality evaluation contains parsing all the reference translations offline using the CoreNLP, extracting dependency n-grams and extending, forming the matching patterns, matching in the candidate translation and calculating the final quality score.

Dependency N-grams Evaluation. We implement the evaluation on three levels: system, document and sentence. Pearson coefficient between dependency n-gram score and human score on system level is shown in Table 1, in which *DnGram* denotes dependency n-gram evaluation, *DnGram-ex* for extended dependency n-grams evaluation. We also list the BLEU and NIST score for comparison.

Table 1 shows DnGram and DnGram-ex outperform the baseline accuracy score of BLEU and NIST significantly, 28.5% over BLEU and 12.6% over NIST.

---

[2] http://translate.google.com.
[3] http://fanyi.baidu.com/.
[4] http://www.yeecloud.com/index.

Table 1. Performance of system level evaluation

	BLEU	NIST	Dngram	Dngram-ex
Flu	**0.702**	0.566	0.555	0.469
Acc	0.696	0.794	0.839	**0.894**

On fluency DnGram is as same as NIST but a little lower than BLEU. The main cause may lie in that the number of n-grams in dependency relations is much less than the traditional n-grams, which n usually is set 4, while most of DnGrams are bigrams. Because data sparseness is not so severe as on system level, fluency evaluation can benefit from the continuous words sequences. However Dngrams favors more on the core meanings.

The result on document level is shown in Table 2.

Table 2. Performance of document level evaluation

	BLEU	NIST	Dngram	Dngram-ex
Flu	**0.172**	0.175	**0.190**	0.182
Acc	0.218	0.219	0.219	**0.222**

Table 2 also confirms the advantage of dependency n-gram evaluation on document level.

On segment level, the performance shown in Table 3 is much lower than that on system and document level because of the data sparseness and variability of sentences. Again the dependency n-gram evaluation algorithm outperforms BLEU on all 1797 sentences. We also include the comparison with the work of [6] denoted as *Related*. The good performance still be kept on segment level. We also notice that the gap between BLEU is enlarged on fluency evaluation, which is a promising result.

Table 3. Performance of segment level evaluation

	BLEU	Related	Dngram-ex
Flu	0.203	0.161	**0.213**
Acc	0.245	0.256	**0.257**

5   Conclusion and Future Work

We applied the dependency n-grams which carrying the core meanings of a sentence to evaluate the quality of machine translation on Chinese medical data. Our work is different with related researches in that we did not apply parser to faulty machine translations. The extracted dependency n-grams are extended according to linguistic rules and implemented in matching patters to capture more semantic similarities between the candidate translation and references. The efficiency of the evaluation is higher since the number of dependency n-grams is much lower than the enumerated n-grams. Furthermore noises introduced by parsing machine translation are significantly reduced.

In future work, we will further explore the method of dependency n-grams extension to better capture the various expression of translations. Also we will incorporate medical domain knowledge into quality evaluation.

References

1. Chen, B., Cherry, C.: A systematic comparison of smoothing techniques for sentence-level BLEU. In: ACL 2014, p. 362 (2014)
2. Cohen, J., et al.: A coefficient of agreement for nominal scales. Educ. Psychol. Measur. **20**(1), 37–46 (1960)
3. Doddington, G.: Automatic evaluation of machine translation quality using n-gram co-occurrence statistics. In: Proceedings of the second international conference on Human Language Technology Research, pp. 138–145 (2002)
4. Lin, C.Y., Och, F.J.: ORANGE: a method for evaluating automatic evaluation metrics for machine translation. In: Proceedings of the 20th International Conference on Computational Linguistics, ACL, pp. 501–507 (2004)
5. Liu, D., Gildea, D.: Syntactic features for evaluation of machine translation. In: Proceedings of the ACL Workshop on Intrinsic and Extrinsic Evaluation Measures for Machine Translation and/or Summarization, pp. 25–32 (2005)
6. Owczarzak, K., van Genabith, J., Way, A.: Labelled dependencies in machine translation evaluation. In: Proceedings of the Second Workshop on Statistical Machine Translation, pp. 104–111. Association for Computational Linguistics (2007)
7. Papineni, K., Roukos, S., Ward, T., et al.: BLEU: a method for automatic evaluation of machine translation. In: Proceedings of the 40th Annual Meeting on Association for Computational Linguistics, ACL, pp. 311–318 (2002)
8. Sidorov, G., Velasquez, F., Stamatatos, E., Gelbukh, A., Chanona-Hernández, L.: Syntactic n-grams as machine learning features for natural language processing. Expert Syst. Appl. **41**(3), 853–860 (2014)
9. Ye, Y., Zhou, M., Lin, C.Y.: Sentence level machine translation evaluation as a ranking problem: one step aside from BLEU. In: Proceedings of the Second Workshop on Statistical Machine Translation, pp. 240–247. Association for Computational Linguistics (2007)
10. Ying, L., Yumei, Z.: Lexis in chinese-english translation of drug package inserts: corpus-based error analysis and its translation strategies. Int. J. Biomed. Sci. IJBS **6**(4), 344 (2010)

A Method of Electronic Medical Record Similarity Computation

Ziping He[1], Jijiang Yang[1(✉)], Qing Wang[1], and Jianqiang Li[2]

[1] Research Institute of Information Technology, Tsinghua University, Beijing, China
hzp14@mails.tsinghua.edu.cn, {yangjijiang,qing.wang}@tsinghua.edu.cn
[2] School of Software Engineering, Beijing University of Technology, Beijing, China
lijianqiang@bjut.edu.cn

Abstract. With the development of electronic healthcare, more and more medical institutions begin to use the information system to manage their patient's health records as well as other healthcare data. Electronic medical records (EMR) contain the patient's personal information, medical history, clinical examination, treatment process, and other information, which have large research value. Today, enormous number of electronic medical records accumulated through the hospital information system all over the world. Analyzing these EMRs can effectively assist doctors in clinical decision-making, provide data support for clinical research as well as personalized healthcare service for patients. This paper presents a EMR similarity computation system. The system accepts EMRs collected from hospitals as input, go through a series of process, and eventually calculates the similarity of any two EMRs. An diseases classification experiment was designed to illustrate the effectiveness of the method. This system lays the foundation for further analysis of electronic medical records.

Keywords: Electronic health record · Similarity computation · Disease classification · KNN classifier

1 Introduction

With the development informationization process of medicine care, more and more hospitals began to use hospital information system (HIS) to assist themselves in clinical research and hospital management. During the popularization of HIS, the traditional paper-based medical records are gradually replaces by electronic medical records (EMR) because of their easiness to lost and inconvenience of storage. An electronic medical record is a patient's personal health records, including a series of medical and healthcare information of a patient, such as personal information, medical history, patient complaint, progress note, surgical records and hospital record. In the face of accumulating number of EMR, it has become an increasing urgent demand to perform analysis and data mining on EMR in order to get useful information of patients and to assist the healthcare process [1].

© Springer International Publishing AG 2017
C. Xing et al. (Eds.): ICSH 2016, LNCS 10219, pp. 182–191, 2017.
DOI: 10.1007/978-3-319-59858-1_18

Most electronic medical records appeared as semi-structured text. On one hand, though we are shifting from traditional hand-writing medical records to electronic medical records, many medical practitioners are still not used to the latter. On the other hand, with many differences between medical information systems of different hospitals, there are no standard regulations of EMR. The existing electronic medical records contain both structured data, such as patient's age, gender, admission time, etc., and unstructured free texts, such as patient complaints, checkup records, surgical records, etc. The unstructured parts of electronic medical records usually have more information of the patient, and are more difficult to analyze.

Similarity computation is a method to evaluate the similarity between two medical records. General text similarity computation [2] has been applied to many scenarios, such as personalized recommendation of e-commerce websites like Amazon, delivery of advertisements on search engines, etc. In terms of biomedical texts, there has not been much research on similarity computation. The application scenarios of similarity computation of electronic medical records include patient social network, disease sketching, detection of side-effects of medicine, medical quality-control, etc. Compared with the common text similarity computation, the similarity computation of electronic medical records has unique difficulties and challenges. One of the challenges is that electronic medical record contains a large number of biomedical terminologies, which must be concerned in order to accurately calculate similarity. On the other hand, electronic medical records are very sensitive to negative expressions, which should be recognized to perform accurate computation.

2 Related Work

Although there have been plenty studies on data mining of biomedical texts [3–9], similarity computation of electronic medical record is still a field with limited research on. Research has been conducted based on the Unified Medical Language System (UMLS) [10], which is managed by medical library of the United States. The research of the automatic indexing and similarity computation of

Table 1. Typical structure of electronic medical record

Label	Attribute
Name	Paul
Gender	Male
Date of birth	1933-11-01
Admission date	2015-06-30
...	...
Complaints	(free text)...
Checkup	(free text)...

electronic medical records written in Chinese has not made significant progress. After the introduction of statistical language model the segmentation and POS tagging of Chinese words accuracy have been greatly improved on processing speed and accuracy. There have been pratical Chinese automatic segmentation system, such as ICTCLAS [11] Segmentation System and the Founder Century Segmentation System. But it is still a long way to go to complete an appropriate biomedical corpus and extend the research of automatic segmentation of Chinese (Table 1).

Syntactic negation analysis in natural language analysis can be very complex [12], the scope of negation function must sometimes rely on common sense to judge. Fortunately, the training for medical record writing require direct and clear description of events and issues [13, 14]. Quantitative study also shows that biomedical documents have less lexical ambiguity compared to non-restricted documents. For English, Mutalick et al. [15] has built a Negfinder, which uses a one-token Look-Ahead Left-to-right Rightmost-derivation parser to recognize negative terms from surgical notes and discharge summaries without extracting full syntactic structure (95.7% sensitivity and 91.8% specificity). Meanwhile the author also mentioned that the method can not correctly detect the negative terms which have larger distance from the negative signals than a preset value. Chapman et al. [16] then proposed a more practical method NegEx based on regular expression. The method has a sensitivity of 77%, an accuracy of 84.5% and specificity of 94.5% recognizing negative terms from discharge notes. Huang and Lowe [17] have two ideas above combined and designed a hybrid algorithm of regular expression matching and syntax parsing, achieving very good results from the radiology reports (92.6% sensitivity, 98.6% accuracy and 99.87% specificity).

Rosenbeck, Goeg, Kirstine [18] conducted some cluster analysis on clinical models. Two groups of clinical models, physical examination and other random clinical models, were selected. After preprocessing the clinical models were presented in SNOMED CT terminologies. Two similarity estimation methods and two clustering strategies were applied in the experiment. The best matching algorithm achieved a good result, which provides a powerful tool for the unification and standardization of clinical model.

3   Method

3.1   System Structure

A complete electronic medical record similarity computation system should include three parts as follows: the basic hospital information system, a data warehouse built to support electronic medical record analysis, and an algorithm to calculate similarity of EMRs.

Hospital Information System (HIS) is a computer application system designed to manage and record all the business activities of the hospital. HIS covers both professional activities (such as surgical records and clinical pathway records) and hospital management (such as employee information and quality control, etc.).

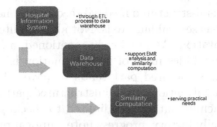

Fig. 1. A complete system of EMR similarity computation

A data warehouse is built to store electronic medical records collected from hospital information system. The main differences between a traditional relational database and a data warehouse are: a data warehouse is built for some analysis purposes, thus is faster in I/O operation than relational databases; a data warehouse is integrated, which means it can extract data from different source databases through an ETL (Extract, Transform and Load) process. Data warehouse also has the characteristics of non-real-time synchronization, large capacity, and preserving historical data, etc. These characteristics make the electronic medical records stored in a data warehouse more suitable for content analyzing and calculating (Fig. 1).

The electronic medical record analysis and similarity computation means analyzing the content of free text in electronic medical records, making EMRs easier to understand by computer, and eventually performing similarity computation. The result of computation can serve multiple practical purposes like detection of medicine side effects and medical healthcare quality control, etc.

3.2 Algorithm

A complete similarity computation algorithm is proposed below. It can be described as Fig. 2 shows.

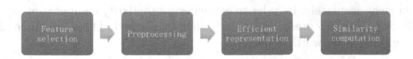

Fig. 2. Algorithm of similarity computation

The input of the algorithm would be a set of EMRs, the element of which records information of patient as a semi-structured document. Patient information includes personal information, history, complaints, diagnosis, progress notes, surgical records and other information.

The output would be similarity of any two EMRs of the EMR set.

(1) Feature selection: Semi-structured medical record documents contain multiple attributes, as many as several hundreds. Not all attributes should be involved in similarity computation. As previously mentioned, a semi-structured electronic medical record hides most of its information hidden in unstructured text field, while the structured part tends to have relatively less information. So we pay more attention to the unstructured part of electronic medical records. Features include but are not limited to checkup record, complaints, medical history, family history, progress note, surgical records and diagnosis.

(2) Preprocess of featured text: The preprocess step include a series of processes like segmentation, stop words filtering, etc., eventually present the text with VSM (Vector Space Model) presentation.

Segmentation. A special step for Chinese electronic medical record. Unlike English and other languages, Chinese sentences don't have natural gap between words. Segmentation technology is quite mature now so won't be discussed here. There are also plenty of open-source segmentation system available. After this step, the text is transformed into a word sequence.

Stop words filtering. Stop words are some words filtered out before natural language processing, in order to save storage space and improve searching efficiency in information retrieval. Common stop words include punctuation and auxiliary words.

Final step is to transform a word sequence to a VSM vector, i.e.:

$$d_j = \{w_{j1}, w_{j2}, ..., w_{jN}\}, j = 1, 2, .., m$$

where N represents the number of words in the dictionary D, which is a set of all words in document set $\mathcal{D}$. Each dimension of the vector represents whether a specific word appeared in the document. For example, $w_i = 0$ means the ith word does not exit in document d_j, and $w_i = 1$ means otherwise. m is the number of documents of the document set $\mathcal{D}$.

(3) More Efficient Document Presentation: The disadvantages of VSM are obvious: document is turn into a high-dimensional sparse vector without considering the semantic importance of words. Thus a VSM vector can not represent a document accurately. In order to get accurate similarity computation results, a better form of representing a document is required. There are three kinds of representation worth considering:

(a) $TF \times iDF$ representation is a relatively dated choice. Each dimension of the document vector still represents a specific word, but its value is replaced with a $TF \times iDF$ value.

   $TF = n_{ji}/(\sum_j n_{ji})$, where n_{ji} is the number word w_i appears in document d_j. It represents term frequency which gets larger when the specific word appears more times in the document.

   $iDF = \log \frac{m}{1+|\{j:word_i \in d_j\}|}$, where $|\{j : word_i \in d_j\}|$ is the number of documents in which $word_i$ appears. iDF value gets smaller when the specific word appears in more documents, so the importance of common words is lowered.

Finally the value $TF \times iDF$ is used to represent the importance of words in documents.

(b) Latent Semantic Index (LSI) representation [19,20]. The $TF \times iDF$ representation does not reduce the number of dimensions of the document vector. Thus it's still a high-dimensional parse vector. LSI representation is an available method to reduce the number of dimensions of vector, to reduce calculation complexity and improve accuracy. LSI model uses SVD decomposition of matrix to extract topics which best represents characters of the document set. Through the LSI dimension reduction a document is represented in a "topic-weight" form, and is more efficient in calculation.

A $t * d$ dimensional matrix (word-document matrix) X can be decomposed into $X = TSD^T$, where T is a $t * m$ matrix and each column in T is called a left singular vector. S is a $m * m$ dimensional diagonal matrix, in which each value is called a singular value. D is a $d * m$ dimensional matrix and each column in it is called a right singular vector. After the SVD decomposition of X, we keep only K largest singular values of S, and corresponding singular vectors in T and D. The kept singular values and vectors form new lower-dimensional matrices S', T' and D'. The new word-document matrix X' is calculated as: $X' = T'S'D'^T$.

On an incoming document d_q, a low-dimensional vector representation is calculated as: $d'_q = d_q T S^{-1}$.

(c) Latent Dirichlet Allocation (LDA) [21] is a popular text generation mode, which can also be used to document classification. LDA is a three-layer Bayesian network generation model, introducing latent topic variables, and assuming that the latent variables subject to multinomial distribution. The optimized parameters of the text generation model is calculated with the principle of Bayesian estimation.

(4) Similarity computation: After gaining the vector representations of two documents, the similarity is determined by the included angle of them:

$$sim(D_1, D_2) = cos(\theta_{D_1, D_2}) = \frac{D_1 \cdot D2}{\|D_1\|\|D_2\|}$$

4   Experiment

4.1   Evaluation Criteria Problem of Computation Results

The similarity between the two electronic medical records can be calculated through the algorithm above, but it can not be evaluated whether the calculation results are accurate or not. One possible evaluation method is to let the medical expert manually evaluate calculation results. This method is too time-consuming and costs too much manpower, also very difficult to perform when the document set gets huge. What's more, different experts may have different opinions on evaluation. Due to the lack of direct evaluation methods, an indirect evaluation method is proposed.

Consider a classification problem to recognize a specific disease using EMRs. There is a EMR set $\mathcal{D}$ and a corresponding label set $\mathcal{Y}$, where $\forall d_i \in \mathcal{D}$ has the label y_i. The label means whether the diagnose in the EMR is the specific disease or not. In order to perform classification in $\mathcal{D}$, the process can be concluded as three simple steps below:

1. determine the training and testing set.
2. train a classifier.
3. test the accuracy using testing set.

The training process involves using a specific distance measure to represent the distance between vectors, such as Euclidean distance and Manhattan distance. Here the similarity computation result can be used as a distance measure. If it shows a better result of classification problem when similarity is used as distance measure, it indicates the similarity calculation works.

4.2   Experiment Design

A set of 76,071 EMRs for experiment are provided by a hospital in Beijing City. The EMRs are stored as semi-structured xml documents. The number of words in the electronic medical record is shown in Fig. 3.

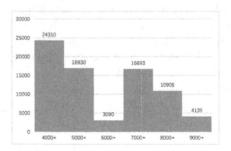

Fig. 3. Distribution of EMRs

We can see more than half of the EMRs are relatively small, due to a lack of free text sections. Therefore, the analysis should be focused on EMRs with more words, especially the 15,408 of which with more than 8,000 words.

In order to perform a classification experiment, 94 EMRs were selected as positive samples, the patients of which were all diagnosed to have lumbar disc protrusion; and 200 randomly chosen EMRs as negative samples. A 4-fold validation method was used in training process. As a preliminary experiment, a KNN classifier was chosen (K = 5).

Two different distance measures were used to train the KNN classifier. One is the Euclidean distance of the document vectors, $\sum_{m=1}^{N} |w_{im} - w_{jm}|^2$. The other

Table 2. Classification accuracy

Distance measure	Classification accuracy
$\sum_{m=1}^{M} |x_{im} - x_{jm}|^2$	0.8946
$1/sim_{(i,j)}$	0.9388

is reciprocal of similarity calculated with the proposed algorithm, $1/sim_{(i,j)}$. The classification result is shown in Table 2.

When K value is changed in training process, the accuracy changed as Fig. 4 shows.

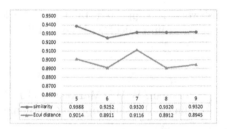

	5	6	7	8	9
similarity	0.9388	0.9252	0.9320	0.9320	0.9320
Ecul distance	0.9014	0.8911	0.9116	0.8912	0.8945

Fig. 4. Experiment results when K changed

As we can see, the classification accuracy is improved after the using reciprocal of the similarity as distance measure, which indicates that calculated similarity can better represent actual similarity of EMRs.

5   Conclusion and Discusstion

Experiments showed that using the similarity as distance measure can effectively improve the accuracy of the disease classification problem, which indicates that the similarity computation of EMRs is an effective method to estimate how similar two EMRs are. The current algorithm is a basic version, and there are certain improvement to be made.

In order to perform more accurate EMR analysis, it is essential to conduct semantic analysis on medical record texts. Different from general text, electronic medical records contain a large number terminologies in biomedical field, which must be specially considered when conducting semantic analysis. There are a number of authoritative corpus of biomedical field, such as SNOMED CT. But due to potential non-standard writing in electronic medical records, the corpus does not completely solve the problem.

One of the ideas to be considered is manual annotation. Manual annotation can effectively solve the problem of identification of terminologies in EMRs. But is costly, and it is difficult to guarantee the accuracy of annotation if done by non-professional personnel.

Another problem is negative expression. EMRs are highly sensitive on negative expressions. For example the terms "fever" and "no fever" represent the exactly opposite meaning in EMRs, but would be considered similar in most similarity calculation methods.

To solve the problem of negative expression, a negative term recognition must be done before further processing. Luckily most EMRs follow strict writing rules, which made possible patterns to recognize negative expressions. However, considering different levels of education and medical training a healthcare provider may accept, there are still challenges in recognizing negative expressions in electronic medical records and more accurate similarity computation.

Acknowledgment. This work is supported by China National Key Technology Research and Development Program project with no. 2013BAH05F02.

References

1. Demner-Fushman, D., Chapman, W.W., McDonald, C.J.: What can natural language processing do for clinical decision support? J. Biomed. Inf. **42**(5), 760–772 (2009)
2. Islam, A., Inkpen, D.: Semantic text similarity using corpus-based word similarity and string similarity. ACM Trans. Knowl. Disc. Data (TKDD) **2**(2), 10 (2008)
3. Mathur, S., Dinakarpandian, D.: Finding disease similarity based on implicit semantic similarity. J. Biomed. Inf. **45**(2), 363–371 (2012)
4. Pedersen, T., Pakhomov, S.V., Patwardhan, S., Chute, C.G.: Measures of semantic similarity and relatedness in the biomedical domain. J. Biomed. Inf. **40**(3), 288–299 (2007)
5. Pedersen, T., Pakhomov, S., McInnes, B., Liu, Y.: Measuring the similarity and relatedness of concepts in the medical domain: Ihi 2012 tutorial overview. In: Proceedings of the 2nd ACM SIGHIT International Health Informatics Symposium, pp. 879–880. ACM (2012)
6. Hersh, W., Mailhot, M., Arnott-Smith, C., Lowe, H.: Selective automated indexing of findings and diagnoses in radiology reports. J. Biomed. Inf. **34**(4), 262–273 (2001)
7. Dong, H., Hussain, F.K.: Semantic service matchmaking for digital health ecosystems. Knowl. Based Syst. **24**(6), 761–774 (2011)
8. SáNchez, D., Batet, M.: Semantic similarity estimation in the biomedical domain: an ontology-based information-theoretic perspective. J. Biomed. Inf. **44**(5), 749–759 (2011)
9. García, M.M., Allones, J.L.I., Hernández, D.M., Iglesias, M.J.T.: Semantic similarity-based alignment between clinical archetypes and snomed CT: an application to observations. Int. J. Med. Inf. **81**(8), 566–578 (2012)
10. Lindberg, D.A., Humphreys, B.L., McCray, A.T.: The unified medical language system. Methods Inf. Med. **32**(4), 281–291 (1993)
11. Zhang, H.-P., Yu, H.-K., Xiong, D.-Y., Liu, Q.: HHMM-based Chinese lexical analyzer ICTCLAS. In: Proceedings of the Second SIGHAN Workshop on Chinese Language Processing, vol. 17, pp. 184–187. Association for Computational Linguistics (2003)

12. Jiang, Y., Zhang, X., Tang, Y., Nie, R.: Feature-based approaches to semantic similarity assessment of concepts using wikipedia. Inf. Process. Manage. **51**(3), 215–234 (2015)
13. Ruch, P., Baud, R., Geissbuhler, A., Rassinoux, A.-M.: Comparing general and medical texts for information retrieval based on natural language processing: an inquiry into lexical disambiguation. Stud. Health Technol. Inf. **1**, 261–265 (2001)
14. McInnes, B.T., Pedersen, T.: Evaluating measures of semantic similarity and relatedness to disambiguate terms in biomedical text. J. Biomed. Inf. **46**(6), 1116–1124 (2013)
15. Mutalik, P.G., Deshpande, A., Nadkarni, P.M.: Use of general-purpose negation detection to augment concept indexing of medical documents. J. Am. Med. Inf. Assoc. **8**(6), 598–609 (2001)
16. Chapman, W.W., Bridewell, W., Hanbury, P., Cooper, G.F., Buchanan, B.G.: A simple algorithm for identifying negated findings and diseases in discharge summaries. J. Biomed. Inf. **34**(5), 301–310 (2001)
17. Huang, Y., Lowe, H.J.: A novel hybrid approach to automated negation detection in clinical radiology reports. J. Am. Med. Inf. Assoc. **14**(3), 304–311 (2007)
18. Gøeg, K.R., Cornet, R., Andersen, S.K.: Clustering clinical models from local electronic health records based on semantic similarity. J. Biomed. Inf. **54**, 294–304 (2015)
19. Dumais, S.T.: Latent semantic analysis. Ann. Rev. Inf. Sci. Technol. **38**(1), 188–230 (2004)
20. Hofmann, T.: Probabilistic latent semantic indexing. In: Proceedings of the 22nd Annual International ACM SIGIR Conference on Research and Development in Information Retrieval, pp. 50–57. ACM (1999)
21. Blei, D.M., Ng, A.Y., Jordan, M.I.: Latent dirichlet allocation. J. Mach. Learn. Res. **3**, 993–1022 (2003)

Heart Rate Variability (HRV) Biofeedback After Stroke Improves Self-regulation of Autonomic Nervous System During Cognitive Stress

Xin Li[1,2], Dechun Sang[1,2(✉)], Yan Zhang[3], Bo Zhang[3], and Chunxiao Xing[3]

[1] School of Rehabilitation Medicine, Capital Medical University, Bejing, China
horsebackdancing@sina.com, sdcl2663@126.com
[2] China Rehabilitation Research Center, Bejing, China
[3] Tsinghua National Laboratory for Information Science and Technology, Department of Computer Science and Technology, Research Institute of Information Technology, Tsinghua University, Beijing, China
zhang-yan14@mails.tsinghua.edu.cn,
bozhang31@sina.com, xingcx@tsinghua.edu.cn

Abstract. Objective: This study aims to investigate the self-regulation of the autonomic nervous system following the cognitive stress tests after Heart Rate Variability (HRV) biofeedback therapy in post-stroke depression (PSD) patients. Methods: Twenty-four patients with PSD were randomly divided into feedback and control groups. Feedback patients were given HRV biofeedback therapy, while the control patients only received relaxation therapy without feedback signal. HRV parameters were tracked during the cognitive stress test in quiet baseline state, cognitive stress state, and resting state, to compare the therapeutic effects of the two groups, before and after treatment. Results: Under the stress conditions, LF of both groups increased, but there were significant differences in the increasing rate (P = 0.02): LF of the feedback group increased slowly, while that of the control group increased rapidly. HRs of both groups increased during the second cognitive test, with HR increasing slowly in the feedback group and faster in the control group (P = 0.05). After rest, the HR of the feedback group decreased significantly faster than that of the control group (P = 0.05). HF of the both group increased during the stress test but showed no significant difference. Conclusion: In this paper, we show that during the cognitive stress test, patients that have received HRV biofeedback therapy can achieve a dynamic balance between sympathetic and parasympathetic nerves by reducing sympathetic sensibility, which improved patients' adaptive capacity to cope with their internal physiological environment and external environmental pressures.

Keywords: Heart rate variability · Biofeedback · Stroke · Self-regulation · Stress test

© Springer International Publishing AG 2017
C. Xing et al. (Eds.): ICSH 2016, LNCS 10219, pp. 192–204, 2017.
DOI: 10.1007/978-3-319-59858-1_19

1 Introduction

The correlation between stress and health/diseases has received increasing attention since the biopsychosocial medical model was proposed in 1970 [1]. Strokes, with high mortality and morbidity, can cause serious harm to the human body. Many stroke patients, affected by psychological, physical and social factors, tend to have mental health problems, often associated with post-stroke depression (PSD) [2]. Without timely and effective self-regulation, the somatic symptoms in patients may get worse under such social and family stressor events, which seriously influences the recovery of neurological function, delays the time for functional recovery, affects patients' quality of life, and imposes a heavy burden on individual patients, family, and society. The stress-induced emotional reactions are closely related to the autonomic nervous activity. The autonomic nervous system can be divided into sympathetic and parasympathetic branches. Emotional reactions are often accompanied by functional changes in the sympathetic and parasympathetic nervous systems. Heart rate variability (HRV) is a simple and effective method to evaluate parasympathetic/sympathetic balance. The frequency domain measures of HRV are divided into different frequency bands based on the heart rate fluctuations, wherein high frequency (HF) reflects parasympathetic activity, low frequency (LF) mainly reflects sympathetic activity, and the ratio of the two (LF/HF) reflects sympathetic and parasympathetic activity in emotional reactions [3].

Self-regulation is a human capacity that allows humans to alter or inhibit their thinking, emotions, and impulsive or explicit behavior. It is closely related to both physical and mental health indexes. Recently, researchers have noted that HRV can be used as a biological indicator of self-regulation [4, 5]. There are individual differences in self-regulation; and a high resting HRV is considered to be associated with health behavior. For example, people with higher HRV can use adaptive emotional regulation and coping strategies to achieve better results in cognitive and attention tasks and have better impulse control. Since there is growing evidence that HRV can be used as a biological indicator of self-regulation, is it possible to use biofeedback therapy to improve HRV to help post-stroke depression patients have higher HRV and thereby improve their self-regulation ability to cope with stressors?

Heart rate variability (HRV) biofeedback requires patients to synchronize fluctuations in breathing and heart rate with slow abdominal breathing (about 5.5 to 6 times per minute, i.e., at the resonance frequency of 0.1 Hz), which maximizes HRV [6]. HRV takes LF as the feedback indicator. It improves psychophysiological indicators and clinical symptoms, especially for those psychosomatic diseases associated with reduced HRV and autonomic dysfunction. HRV biofeedback can reduce substance abuse [6] and food addiction [7] for patients with posttraumatic stress disorder. Li et al. [8] have done a lot of research on the effect of HRV biofeedback therapy in PSD patients and found it has a therapeutic effect, improving patients' mood, sleep, and HRV indexes, but they mentioned little about coping with stressors. In this study, using various cognitive tests as stressors, we discuss the physiological arousal effect that HRV biofeedback has on stress, and our results provide strong evidence for implementing stress intervention during negative events.

2   Methods

2.1   Patient Selection

Subjects of the study were recruited among the rehabilitation inpatients in Beijing Bo Ai Hospital from February 2013 to May 2014. Eligible subjects were selected according to the inclusion criteria and exclusion criteria used in Li et al. [8]. The study protocol was approved by the Ethics Committee of Beijing Bo Ai Hospital and written informed consent was obtained from all participants.

2.2   Procedure and Randomization

Patients enrolled in the experiment were divided into feed back and control groups according to the randomized controlled trials table. All subjects received regular rehabilitation treatments including physical therapy, psychotherapy, and medication (fluoxetine, 20 mg daily). The patients in the feedback group were given additional HRV biofeedback treatments (30 min each time, 3 times/week for 4–6 weeks, and 10 times as a course), following the protocol of Lehrer et al. [9]. The patients in the control group received relaxation therapy without a feedback signal to guide them in breathing quietly and staying awake.

The embodiments of the feedback group are based on guidelines of HRV biofeedback therapy [9]. Concrete steps are as follows: (i) Patients take the initiative to adjust the frequency and amplitude of respiration in a relaxed, natural way. They are required to do deep, slow, and controlled abdominal breathing and pursed-lip breathing exercises, which should be relaxed, comfortable, and not too laborious to avoid hyperventilation due to breathing too deeply. Expiratory time should be longer than the inspiratory time. (ii) When patients grasp the essentials of reducing respiratory rate, tell patients that the heart rate is synchronized with breathing, that is, heart rate rises during inspiration and decreases during expiration. Show schematic diagram of heart rate variability and respiratory phase on the screen simultaneously. Guide patients to adjust their breathing pattern to change the diagram of heart rate fluctuations so as to synchronize heart rate with breathing and then increase the amplitude of heart rate fluctuations gradually, which is the basic process of HRV biofeedback. (iii) Once patients learn the self-training breathing pattern, they continue to train at home to strengthen these reflections and improve baroreceptor reflex function to achieve functional balance.

To find the change rules of HRV indexes under stress conditions and to compare the therapeutic effects of the two groups, indexes of HRV, including standard deviation of normal RR intervals (SDNN), HR, low frequency (LF), high frequency (HF), and LF/HF ratio, were tracked by a multi-channel biofeedback instrument in quiet baseline state, stress state, and resting state after stress. Stress cognitive tests are as follows. After placing the detection electrode, first record patient's physiological indexes in his/her natural, quiet state for 3 min to provide a baseline. Then follow the instructions to complete the cognitive stressor tasks, a mental arithmetic test and recall test. Patients are required to complete the tasks quickly and accurately, with each task lasting 3 min while physiological indexes are recorded. There is no break in this stress phase. The rest phase starts after testing, and physiological indexes in the 3 min quiet state are recorded again.

Figure 1 shows the experiment framework.

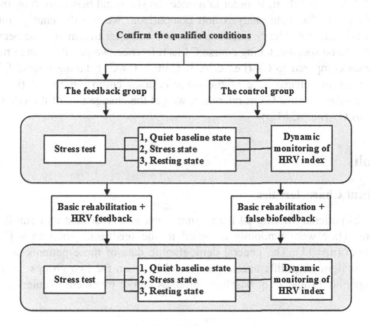

Fig. 1. Experiment framework

2.3   Equipment and Materials

HRV biofeedback training was conducted in the biofeedback and cognitive laboratory of Beijing Bo Ai Hospital. Biofeedback equipment was a VBFB type biofeedback system, named VBFB-3000 (dual display), and was provided by Nanjing Vishee Medical Technology Co., Ltd. The software system used was the Chinese version of BioNeuro Infiniti 5.1. We conducted time- and frequency-domain analysis on the HRV data collected in 3 min increments. We used the fast Fourier transform (FFT) option for the logarithmic conversion of frequency-domain HRV parameters.

The Basic Cognitive Capability Test (Standalone Version 1.0) and its relevant software were used in our stress test. The test had 4 courses in total, namely baseline before stress (course1), cognitive stress phase (course2 for mental arithmetic test and course3 for recall test), and rest phase after stress (course4) in chronological order. To find the change rules of parameters under stress conditions and to compare the therapeutic effects of the two groups, physiological parameter data such as HRV parameters within 3 min were collected during each course.

2.4 Statistical Analysis

We applied SPSS 19.0 for statistical analysis. The change rate of all courses in the stress test was compared using χ^2 test. The stress test can be divided into baseline before stress (course1), cognitive stress phase (course2 for mental arithmetic test and course3 for recall test), and rest phase after stress (course4) in chronological order, that is, C1, C2, C3, C4 for short. In order to reduce the statistical bias caused by individual differences and to facilitate analysis and comparison, we use the change rate of all courses to evaluate the efficacy differences before and after treatment, and between the two groups. To be specific, taking course C1 as reference, we get the change rate of the other courses compared to C1 (i.e., C2/C1, C3/C1, C4/C1); taking course C2 as reference, we get the change rate of the other courses compared to C2 (i.e., C3/C2, C4/C2); and taking course C3 as reference, we get the change rate of the other courses compared to C3 (i.e., C4/C3).

3 Results

3.1 Patient Characteristics

A total of 24 patients meeting all the requirements were recruited and enrolled in the experiment. They were randomly assigned to the feedback group (n = 13) or the control group (n = 11). The general demographic data of these patients are listed in Table 1. No significant differences were found between the two groups in terms of any demographic (Table 1) or baseline variables before treatment (Table 2).

Table 1. Basic characteristics of control and feedback groups

Characteristics	Feedback group (n = 13)	Control group (n = 11)
Age (years), mean ± SD	54.38 ± 13.33	59.64 ± 12.44
Gender, n		
Female	8	3
Male	5	8
Education, n		
Elementary	2	1
High school	4	7
Graduate	7	3
Married, n	13	11
Diagnosis, n		
Infarction	8	6
Hemorrhage	5	5
Effect side, n		
Left	10	6

(*continued*)

Table 1. (*continued*)

Characteristics	Feedback group (n = 13)	Control group (n = 11)
Right	3	5
Course of disease (months), mean ± SD	3.62 ± 2.18	3.36 ± 1.43
Involved part, n		
Parietal	1	2
Temporal	4	5
Prefrontal	5	1
Basal	12	10
Single lesion, n	6	7
Medical history, n		
Hypertension	10	11
Diabetes	3	2
Heart disease	3	0
Hyperlipidemia	4	8
Mood, n		
Depression	3	4
Anxiety	10	7

[a]SD: Standard deviation.

3.2   Changes in LF

From the quiet state (C1) to the beginning of cognitive tests (C2), the LF of both groups increased, but their increasing ratio showed significant differences. Specifically, the LF of the feedback group increased slowly, while that of the control group increased rapidly at a speed nearly 8 times faster than the feedback group. Compared with the control group, the change rate of the feedback group showed no significant difference during and after the test, as shown in Table 2 and Fig. 2.

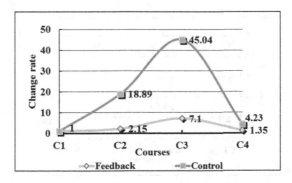

Fig. 2. Change rate of LF in cognitive stress state. The change rate of each course was derived by taking course C1 as reference, and it also applies to the following figures.

3.3 Changes in HF

The HF of both groups increased during test and decreased after test. The trends and change rate of each phase were similar and there were no significant differences between the two groups, as shown in Table 2 and Fig. 3.

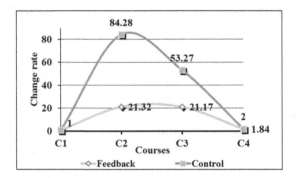

Fig. 3. Change rate of HF in cognitive stress state.

3.4 Changes in HR

From the baseline state (C1) to the completion of the first cognitive stress test (C2), the HR of the feedback group increased, with no significant difference between the two groups. During the second cognitive stress test (C3), the HR of both groups increased, and there were significant differences between the two groups, with the HR increasing slowly in the feedback group and somewhat faster in the control group. Compared with the control group, the feedback group showed no significant difference in the change rate in the above two courses. However, HRs in the feedback group decreased faster than in the control group in the late course the late-course, with final values lower than the baseline level, while that of the control group was still higher than baseline over the same period, as shown in Table 2 and Fig. 4.

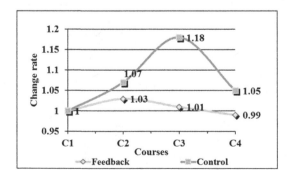

Fig. 4. Change rate of HR in cognitive stress state.

Table 2. The change rate of HRV parameters during stress test ($\bar{x}$, χ^2)

Items	Group	Treatment phase	C2/C1	C3/C1	C4/C1	C3/C2	C4/C2	C4/C3
HR	Feedback group (n = 13)	Before	1.03	1.02	0.91	0.99	0.88	0.89
		After	1.03	1.01* *P = 0.02	0.99* *P = 0.05	0.98	0.96	0.98
	Control group (n = 11)	Before	1.09	1.10	0.91	1.01	0.80	0.83
		After	0.95	1.08	1.02	0.99	0.95	0.95
SDNN	Feedback group (n = 13)	Before	1.89	2.22	1.46	1.18	0.86	0.79
		After	2.47	2.14	1.21	1.22	0.83	0.78
	Control group (n = 11)	Before	2.38	3.58	1.68	1.77	0.61	0.53
		After	5.15	4.73	1.96	1.45	0.46	0.59
LF	Feedback group (n = 13)	Before	12.89	3.53	1.16	1.15	0.61	0.73
		After	2.15* *P = 0.02	7.10	1.35	3.05	2.17	1.79
	Control group (n = 11)	Before	13.78	22.12	5.49	3.69	0.30	0.83
		After	18.89	45.04	4.23	1.73	0.40	0.61
HF	Feedback group (n = 13)	Before	9.31	16.32	4.77	1.60	1.26	1.12
		After	21.32	21.17	1.84	4.39	0.52	0.32
	Control group (n = 11)	Before	17.56	28.40	14.47	4.30	0.47	0.84
		After	84.28	53.27	2.00	4.57	0.19	0.27
LF/HF	Feedback group (n = 13)	Before	2.45	1.08	1.39	0.80	1.84	1.77
		After	0.63	0.44	2.08	0.97	11.7	12.95
	Control group (n = 11)	Before	1.44	1.71	0.76	1.11	0.60	0.97
		After	0.52	0.93	3.27	3.16	13.20	4.60

*P < 0.05, comparison of two groups before and after treatment; SDNN: Standard deviation of normal RR intervals; LF: Low frequency; HF: High frequency; HR: Heart rate.

Table 3. HRV parameters during stress test (mean ± SD)

Items	Group	Treatment Phase	C1	C2	C3	C4
HR (beats/min)	Feedback group (n = 13)	Before	80.20 ± 9.46	82.61 ± 10.90	81.84 ± 14.16	72.98 ± 18.25
		After	79.97 ± 14.28	82.37 ± 3.18	80.77 ± 15.20	79.17 ± 8.91
	Control group (n = 11)	Before	78.87 ± 12.60	85.97 ± 1.19	86.76 ± 1.92	71.77 ± 13.00
		After	74.65 ± 15.30	70.9 ± 8.91	80.62 ± 12.63	76.14 ± 18.25
SDNN (ms)	Feedback group (n = 13)	Before	36.19 ± 24.15	68.40 ± 29.46	80.34 ± 32.05	52.84 ± 15.89
		After	44.62 ± 32.23	110.21 ± 12.82	95.49 ± 35.11	53.99 ± 11.60
	Control group (n = 11)	Before	35.15 ± 35.50	83.66 ± 16.04	125.84 ± 31.88	59.05 ± 13.46
		After	18.22 ± 11.27	93.83 ± 39.71	86.18 ± 17.13	35.71 ± 37.31
LF (ms)	Feedback group (n = 13)	Before	62.18 ± 114.91	801.50 ± 105.56	219.50 ± 90.14	72.13 ± 129.17
		After	273.93 ± 462.78	588.95 ± 332.67	1944.90 ± 87.43	369.81 ± 93.78

(continued)

Table 3. (*continued*)

Items	Group	Treatment Phase	C1	C2	C3	C4
	Control group (n = 11)	Before	77.69 ± 147.72	1070.57 ± 114.95	1718.50 ± 178.09	426.52 ± 102.33
		After	16.36 ± 25.63	309.04 ± 102.70	736.85 ± 68.23	62.20 ± 98.11
HF (ms)	Feedback group (n = 13)	Before	71.31 ± 84.77	663.90 ± 69.07	1163.78 ± 120.21	130.15 ± 47.90
		After	98.80 ± 218.17	2106.42 ± 401.99	2091.60 ± 72.11	181.79 ± 63.19
	Control group (n = 11)	Before	190.56 ± 405.96	3346.23 ± 201.89	5411.90 ± 129.28	2757.40 ± 89.09
		After	23.95 ± 39.93	2018.51 ± 331.01	1275.82 ± 44.91	47.90 ± 71.32
LF/HF	Feedback group (n = 13)	Before	0.97 ± 0.70	2.38 ± 0.28	1.05 ± 0.58	1.35 ± 1.28
		After	8.52 ± 16.66	5.37 ± 1.53	3.75 ± 2.02	17.72 ± 1.87
	Control group (n = 11)	Before	0.82 ± 0.62	1.18 ± 2.38	1.40 ± 3.05	0.62 ± 0.98
		After	2.01 ± 2.19	1.04 ± 1.77	1.87 ± 0.14	6.57 ± 2.00

[a]HR: Heart rate; SDNN: Standard deviation of normal RR intervals; LF: Low frequency; HF: High frequency.

4 Discussion

In 1936 Selye defined the concept of stress as "the non-specific physiological response of the body to any demand" [10]. He also put forward the concept of "general adaptation syndrome" and pointed out that stress was accompanied by a series of body reactions, such as increased heart rate, elevated blood pressure, accelerated breathing, and reduced gastrointestinal motility [11]. Since then, the concept of stress was further developed. Day [12] proposed adopting Selye's (re-worded) definition of stress as "the body's multi-system response to any challenge that overwhelms, or is judged likely to overwhelm, selective homeostatic response mechanisms." Studies have found that psychological stress, depression, and anxiety are associated with disorders of the autonomic nervous system [13, 14]. Patients with different physiological diseases have abnormal autonomic activity, such as cardiovascular disease [15], irritable bowel syndrome [16], migraine [17], and arrhythmia [18]. Therefore it has been proposed that disorders appearing during the adaptation process of autonomic regulation have a negative impact on the body [19]. The subcortical level regulates the physiological stress-induced responses of the autonomic nervous system with bottom-up control, while the psychological stress-induced responses of the autonomic nervous system are regulated by higher-order brain structures such as the prefrontal lobe. Stroke patients' nerve pathways will be affected by the impaired brain function, and the autonomic nervous system will gradually lose its central integration function, resulting in severe damage to the balance between the sympathetic and parasympathetic systems and a decrease in HRV. In addition, limb movement disorders affect patients' ability to control their limbs and take care of themselves. This reduces their capacity to cope with severe and complex stress, often manifested by emotional responses including anxiety and depression, sleep disorders, anergy, easy fatigue, indolence, and rejection of training. It may also induce or aggravate serious diseases such as cardiovascular disease (Table 3).

In this study, we found that the ability of HRV biofeedback to adapt to the external environment changed as follows. Both LF and HF indexes increased rapidly when stress was introduced and decreased during the rest phase. Both sympathetic and parasympathetic activity were increased by cognitive stressors and decreased synchronously after stress. This finding is consistent with that of Berntso, where the response of each branch of the autonomic nervous system is independent of each other and no interaction is found between the sympathetic and parasympathetic nervous system [20, 21]. Mental stress can change the response of the central-peripheral regulatory system [22, 23]. Such changes influence different pathways respectively, leading to long duration or overreaction in the increase or decrease of the sympathetic/parasympathetic nervous system activity of a specific target organ [24]. What's more, the response is lack of adaptability, which can eventually damage patients' health. This study also found significant differences between the low frequency (LF) change rate of both groups (C2/C1: 18.89 and 2.15 respectively, P = 0.02), with LF increasing rapidly in the control group but slowly in the feedback group. LF is jointly modulated by the vagal and sympathetic systems, but it mainly reflects the activity of the sympathetic nervous system. The rapid increase in LF of the control group under stress conditions indicates a relatively or excessively high stress level in patients, manifested by sympathetic hyperactivity in response to stress. After HRV biofeedback training, LF increased slowly in the stress state, showing that HRV biofeedback can reduce the sensitivity of sympathetic nerve function, lower the speed and magnitude of sympathetic activation, and prevent overactivity of the sympathetic system after stress. It is generally recognized that a certain degree of stress level can improve work efficiency. However, sympathetic overactivity is a leading cause of cardiovascular and cerebrovascular diseases. HRV biofeedback can control sympathetic nerve activity effectively, which improves the adaptability of the response and provides necessary conditions for patients to cope with pressure and adapt to the external environment, as well as to quickly regulate their autonomic nervous system. In conclusion, HRV biofeedback can increase the threshold for various stressors, reduce the sensitivity of the sympathetic nerve function, and enhance patients' adaptive capacity to cope with various changes.

This study also showed that HF increased with the appearance of stressors and decreased after stress test. Nolan et al. [25] found that HF increased significantly during the stress and recovery phases in an exercise stress test and considered it to result from the increased vagal tone. Different from the findings reported in their study, our experiment didn't show significant effect of HRV biofeedback on HF, which means that HRV biofeedback doesn't simply enhance the parasympathetic activity to response to cognitive stressors.

Under stress conditions, the heart rate (HR) changes as follows. HR increased during the quiet state and the stress state. It increased rapidly at the beginning; as time goes by, it gradually decreased and was finally down to the baseline level after rest. When coping with stressors after treatment, the HR change rates of the two groups were significantly different (C3/C1: 1.01 and 1.08 respectively, P = 0.02). Although HRs of both groups increased due to the sympathomimetic effect, the HR of the feedback group increased more slowly than that of the control group, which was similar to that of LF. During the resting state after stress, the HR change rates of both groups still showed significant differences (C4/C1: 0.99 and 1.02 respectively, P = 0.05), with the reduced HR speed in the feedback group much more apparent than that in the control group. The final value of HR in the feedback group is down to or even less than the baseline level, while that of the control group was still higher. To sum up, patients were in stress when given stressors; and because of the quick sympathetic system response, manifested by the accelerated HR and increased sympathetic tone, the feedback groups' sympathetic nerve function sensitivity decreased and, therefore, there was no significant increase in HR. The difference in this phase can be explained by changes in LF. After stress, the HR decreased rapidly to the baseline or an even lower level in a relatively short period of time, which shortened the recovery time. As there was no significant difference in the change rate of HR of both groups, it is difficult to explain this with sympathetic-parasympathetic interactions, which are manifested as an increasing parasympathetic tone to cope with sympathetic system. The mechanism may be complicated and further study is required. In a word, HR in the feedback group is around the baseline level with small amplitude from beginning to the end, even under the stress condition, indicating that HRV biofeedback promotes a dynamic equilibrium between individuals' sympathetic and parasympathetic system, enhances their adaptive capacity to cope with various changes, and shortens their recovery time to cope with external environmental pressures.

Many studies have reported that PSD patients show continuous hyperactivity of the hypothalamic-pituitary-adrenal (HPA) axis under stress conditions, which leads to a series of pathophysiological changes. If glucocorticoid increases repeatedly or persistently, hippocampal glucocorticoid receptor down-regulation occurs, which will damage the glucocorticoid negative feedback regulation, resulting in continuous activity of the HPA axis, further damage of the hippocampus, and more serious mood disorders. With HPA hyperfunction, the increased glucocorticoid degrades plasma tryptophan by inducing liver tryptophan pyrrolase, resulting in central tryptophan deficiency and low 5-hydroxytryptamine (5-HT) synthesis rates [26]. Under long-term stress, this can lead to long-term release and even depletion of 5-HT and norepinephrine (NE), further aggravating mood disorders [27]. We suggest that, when coping with stressors in cognitive testing, HRV biofeedback produces effects by regulating the HPA axis function, decreasing the glucocorticoid level, reducing sympathetic activity, and continuing the autonomic nervous system balance. This study reveals that the virtuous self-regulation of biofeedback plays a role not only in the respiratory feedback operation, but also in the intervals between treatments where no feedback signal is given, or even in the process of stress resistance, which is of significant importance for the functional recovery of rehabilitation patients. Lehrer [28, 29] thinks that HRV biofeedback has a long-term efficacy on the increase of baroreflex tension, which may be related to the fact that the baroreflex promotes there modeling and regeneration of nerve cells. Once patients master breathing techniques in HRV biofeedback and realize its effect on mood improvement and stress event management, they will repeat the intensive training spontaneously and thereby achieve the ability to counter or adapt to internal physiological and external environmental pressures. This in-depth study of neuro immunology mechanisms of HRV biofeedback provides a broader view for treatment of PSD.

We presumed to find the objective, single index of HRV to evaluate the data generated by HRV biofeedback when coping with stressors. However, only LF and HR were different between the two groups. As these indexes were innervated by both sympathetic and parasympathetic system, it is difficult to derive the patterns of autonomic nervous activity. Research about the response patterns of the autonomic nervous system under stress conditions requires consummation data, enlarged samples, and strict control of unrelated factors to further clarify the mechanisms. The stressors in our study are psychological pressures caused by cognitive tests rather than common fear and anxiety, that is, emotional stress and exercise stress. In future work, we can consummate the type and intensity of stressors to better stimulate real-life stress and clarify the patterns of autonomic nervous activity under different types of stress.

5 Conclusion

In this paper, we show that physiological arousal effect of HRV biofeedback therapy helps PSD patients have higher HRV and thereby improve their self-regulation ability to cope with stressors by reducing sympathetic sensibility, which shortens patients' time to recovery from external environmental pressures and enhances their adaptive capacity to cope with various changes. HRV biofeedback is a beneficial adjuvant treatment for patients after stroke.

References

1. Liu, X., Liang, B.Y.: The relationship among mental arithmetic stress, trait anxiety and coping style. Stud. Psychol. Behav. **6**(1), 30–37 (2008)
2. Yang, M.M.: Relationship among depression, anxiety and possible factors in post stroke patients: 510 cases report. Chin. J. Rehabil. Theory Pract. **2**, 498–500 (2006)
3. Zhang, W.C., Yan, K.L., Lu, Y.Q., Zhang, D., Hong, J., Yuan, L.Z., et al.: The effect of different psychological stressors on responses of sympathetic and parasympathetic nervous systems. **39**(2), 285–291 (2007)
4. Segerstro, S.C., Nes, L.S.: Heart rate variability reflects self-regulatory strength, effort, and fatigue. Psychol. Sci. **18**(3), 275–281 (2007)
5. Wang, W., Chen, H.: Heart rate variability is a biomarker of self-regulation. Psychology **1**, 16–19 (2015)
6. Zucker, T.L., Samuelson, K.W., Muench, F., Greenberg, M.A., Gevirtz, R.N.: The effects of respiratory sinus arrhythmia biofeedback on heart rate variability and post traumatic stress disorder symptoms: a pilot study. Appl. Psychophysiol. Biofeedback **34**(2), 135–143 (2009)
7. Meule, A., Freund, R., Skirde, A.K., Vögele, C., Kübler, A.: Heart rate variability biofeedback reduces food cravings in high food cravers. Appl. Psychophysiol. Biofeedback **37**(4), 241–251 (2012)
8. Li, X., Zhang, T., Song, L.P., Zhang, Y., Zhang, G.G., Xing, C.X., et al.: Effects of heart rate variability biofeedback therapy on patients with post stroke depression: a case study. Chin. Med. J. **128**(18), 2542–2545 (2015)

9. Lehrer, P.M., Vaschillo, E., Vaschillo, B., Lu, S.E., Eckberg, D.L., Edelberg, R.: Heart rate variability biofeedback increases barore flex gain and peak expiratory flow. Psychosom. Med. **65**(5), 796–805 (2003)

10. Selye, H.: A syndrome produced by diverse nocuous agents. Nature **138**, 32 (1936)

11. Selye, H.: The general adaptation syndrome and the diseases of adaptation. J. Clin. Endocrinol. Metab. **6**(2), 117–230 (1946)

12. Day, T.A.: Defining stress as a prelude to mapping its neurocircuitry: no help from all ostasis. Prog. Neuropsychopharmacol. Biol. Psychiatry **29**(8), 1195–1200 (2005)

13. Hughes, J.W., Stoney, C.M.: Depressed mood is related to high frequency heart rate variability during stressors. Psychosomat. Med. **62**(6), 796–803 (2000)

14. Stein, P.K., Carney, R.M., Freedland, K.E., Skala, J.A., Jaffe, A.S., Kleiger, R.E., et al.: Severe depression is associated with markedly reduced heart rate variability in patients with stable coronary heart disease. J. Psychosom. Res. **48**(4–5), 493–500 (2000)

15. Vale, S.: Psychosocial stress and cardiovascular diseases. Postgrad. Med. J. **81**(957), 429–435 (2005)

16. Mawdsley, J.E., Rampton, D.S.: Psychological stress in IBD: new insights into pathogenic and the rapeutic implications. Gut **54**(10), 1481–1491 (2005)

17. Davis, P.A., Holm, J.E., Myers, T.C., Suda, K.T.: Stress, headache, and physiological disregulation: a time-series analysis of stress in the laboratory. Headache **38**, 116–121 (1998)

18. Esler, M.: The autonomic nervous system and cardiac arrhythmias. Clin. Auton. Res. **2**(2), 133–135 (1992)

19. Depue, R.A., Monroe, S.M.: Conceptualization and measurement of human disorder in life stress research: the problem of chronic disturbance. Psychol. Bull. **99**(1), 36–51 (1986)

20. Berntson, G.G., Cacioppo, J.T., Quigley, K.S.: Autonomic determinism: the modes of autonomic control, the doctrine of autonomic space, and the laws of autonomic constraint. Psychol. Rev. **98**(4), 459–487 (1991)

21. Berntson, G.G., Cacioppo, J.T., Binkley, P.F., Uchino, B.N., Quigley, K.S., Fieldstone, A.: Autonomic cardiac control: III. psychological stress and cardiac response in autonomic space as revealed by pharmacological blockades. Psychophysiology **31**(6), 599–608 (1994)

22. Bremner, J.D., Randall, P., Vermetten, E., Staib, L., Bronen, R.A., Mazure, C., et al.: Magnetic resonance imaging based measurement of hippocampal volume in posttraumatic stress disorders related to childhood physical and emotional abuse a preliminary report. Biol. Psychiatry **41**(1), 23–32 (1997)

23. Fuchs, E., Uno, H., Flügge, G.: Chronic psychosocial stress induces morphologic alterations in hippocampal pyramidal neurons of the treeshrew. Brain Res. **673**(2), 275–282 (1995)

24. Mayer, E.A.: Emerging disease model for functional gastrointestinal disorders. Am. J. Med. **107**(5A), 12S–19S (1999)

25. Nolan, R.P., Kamath, M.V., Floras, J.S., Stanley, J., Pang, C., Picton, P., et al.: Heart rate variability biofeedback as a behavioral neurocardiac intervention to enhance vagal heart control. Am. Heart J. **149**(6), 1137 (2005)

26. Bigger, J.T., Fleiss, J.L., Rolnitzky, L.M., Steinman, R.C.: The ability of several short-term measures of RR variability to predict mortality after myocardial infarction. Circulation **88**(3), 927–934 (1993)

27. Azmitia, E.C., Whitaker-Azmitia, P.M.: Awakening the sleeping giant: anatomy and plasticity of the brain serotonergic system. J. Clin. Phychiatry **Suppl**, 4–16 (1991)

28. Lehrer, P.M., Vaschillo, E., Vaschillo, B., Lu, S.E., Scardella, A., Siddique, M., et al.: Biofeedback treatment for asthma. Chest **126**(2), 352–361 (2004)

29. Lehrer, P.M.: Applied psychophysiology: beyond the boundaries of biofeedback (mending a wall, a brief history of our field, and applications to control of the muscles and cardiorespiratory systems). Appl. Psychophysiol. Biofeedback **28**(4), 291–304 (2003)

A Medical Image Retrieval Algorithm Based on DFT Encryption Domain

Chunyan Zhang, Jingbing Li[✉], Shuangshuang Wang,
Yucong Duan, Mengxing Huang, and Daoheng Duan

College of Information Science and Technology,
Hainan University, Haikou, China
13739198205@163.com, wangssll16@163.com,
huangmx09@163.com, ddh_335@163.com,
jingbingli2008@hotmail.com, duanyucong@hotmail.com

Abstract. The medical image needs to be encrypted before storing in cloud platform to protect against leaking the personal private information of medical image. And we expect the encrypted medical image can be retrieved automatically in cloud computing platform, but traditional medical image retrieval is based on the visual feature, which is difficult to identify with the naked eye after encryption. In this paper, we propose an algorithm with strong robustness— medical image retrieval algorithm based on DFT encryption domain. We encrypt the image in frequency domain and extract its feature vector to establish a feature database, and then automatically compute the NC (Normalized Cross Correlation Coefficient, NC) between the feature vector of the image to be retrieved and each one stored in the feature database. Finally, the corresponding encrypted image with the greatest value of NC is returned. The experimental results show that this algorithm has ideal ability to resist the conventional attack, such as interference of Gaussian noise, JPEG compressing and median filtering, and geometric attack, such as rotation, scaling, translation, cutting.

Keywords: DFT encryption domain · Encrypted medical image retrieval · Feature vector · NC · Robustness

1 Introduction

Nowadays computer imaging and database techniques play an important role in medical field, which leads to the huge amount of digital images with a wide variety of image modalities, such as Computed Tomography (CT), Magnetic Resonance (MR), X-ray and ultrasound images [1]. With wide use of cloud platform, more and more images are stored in an outsourced way (e.g. Cloud storage platform) to reduce exploitation cost and share resources conveniently. Cloud platform can also form an exchange platform that all healthcare organizations use.

For privacy-preserving purposes, sensitive medical images need to be encrypted before outsourcing, which makes the CBIR technologies in plain-text domain to be unavailable. CBIR need to extracted the feature vector, such as texture [3], shape [4], color [5], from the encrypted medical image stored in cloud, but after using traditional

© Springer International Publishing AG 2017
C. Xing et al. (Eds.): ICSH 2016, LNCS 10219, pp. 205–216, 2017.
DOI: 10.1007/978-3-319-59858-1_20

ways of encryption, such as DES, IDEA, AES and so on, the visual feature of encrypted images are difficult to be identified, so it is a problem urgent to be resolved that doctors and other relevant researchers how to find the required image accurately and rapidly from a huge amount of encrypted medical images stored in cloud computing.

Homomorphic encryption [6–8] is a novel way, which allows us to perform other operations on the encrypted image without decryption, and the result is equivalent to the same operation on a non-encrypted image, for example, In [9], Erkin et al. proposed the privacy-preserving biometric face recognition protocol based on additive homomorphic encryption where a query image is sent homomorphically encrypted to the server. And biometric recognition by adopting the additive homomorphic encryption technique was also mentioned in [10–12]. The operation of image encryption and retrieval can be carried out in spatial domain and frequency domain. When the medical image suffers the slight geometry attack such as partial distortion, the pixels values will suddenly change, and the visual features extracted in the space domain will obviously mutate. In order to extract the medical image feature more accurately for improving the retrieval efficiency, a sort of novel feature called "frequency layer feature" [13].

In this paper, we propose an algorithm for medical image retrieval based on DFT transform and Logistic Chaotic Map Encryption. This method combines the visual feature with encryption technology to protect sensitive information of medical image and retrieve required image rapidly and accurately after conventional attacks and geometric attacks. It shortens the time of encryption and retrieving, and improves efficiency and robustness.

2   Fundamental Theory

2.1   Discrete Fourier Transform (DFT)

The mapping relationship between time domain and frequency domain of Discrete Fourier Transform (DFT) can be fully reflected in a cycle. Suppose there is a M × N medical image, the following formula can be used to performed DFT transform.

$$F(u,v) = \sum_{x=0}^{M-1} \sum_{y=0}^{N-1} f(x,y) \cdot e^{-j2\pi xu/M} e^{-j2\pi yv/N} \tag{1}$$

$$u = 0, 1, \ldots, M-1 \; ; \; v = 0, 1, \ldots, N-1$$

The formula of IDFT transform is as following:

$$f(x,y) = \frac{1}{MN} \sum_{u=0}^{M-1} \sum_{v=0}^{N-1} F(u,v) e^{j2\pi\left(\frac{ux}{M} + \frac{vy}{N}\right)} \tag{2}$$

$$x = 0, 1, \ldots, M-1 \; ; \; y = 0, 1, \ldots, N-1$$

In which, f(x, y) corresponds the value of sampling point (x, y) of medical image in spatial domain, F(u, v) matches the value of DFT coefficients at point (u, v) in frequency domain. Digital image usually used pixel square, that is M = N.

2.2 Logistic Map

Chaos is a similar random process in a deterministic system. One dimensional logistic mapping is a very simple chaos mapping from mathematical form, which is extremely sensitive to the initial value. It is widely used in the field of secure communication, and its mathematical formula is as following:

$$x_{k+1} = \mu x_k (1 - x_k) \tag{3}$$

Where $0 \le \mu \le 4$ is growth parameters, $x_k \in (0, 1)$ is the variables in system. k is the number of iterations. The petty change to the initial value will lead to significant difference in the chaotic sequence, so the above sequence is an idea key sequence. In this paper, $\mu = 4$.

3   The Algorithm Process

3.1   Encryption Algorithm of Medical Image

Figure 1 is the flow chart of medical image encryption. The encryption process is as following:

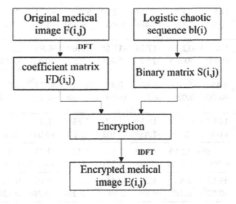

Fig. 1. The flow chart of medical image encryption.

1. Carry out DFT on original medical image F(i, j) to acquire complex coefficient matrix FD(i, j);
2. Set the initial value x_0, and apply logistic map to generate a one-dimensional chaotic sequence bl(i);

3. Define a threshold sign function SI(i), and turn bl(i) into a binary chaotic sequence only contained 1 and −1, construct a binary matrix S(i, j) consistent with medical image size;
4. Do a dot products between the DFT complex coefficient matrix FD(i, j) of medical image and binary matrix S(i, j) to obtain L(i, j);
5. Implement inverse Discrete Fourier Transform (IDFT) on L(i, j) to gain the encrypted image E(i, j);

$$SI(bl(j)) = \begin{cases} 1 & bl(j) \geq 0.5 \\ -1 & bl(j) < 0.5 \end{cases} \tag{4}$$

3.2 Extract the Feature Vector of Encrypted Medical Image to Be Retrieval

Firstly, the encrypted medical image is computed by DFT, obtaining DFT complex coefficient matrix. Then, the first 2 × 4 coefficient matrix ED(1, 1)–ED(1, 4), ED(2, 1)–ED(2, 4) is be chosen (a complex is treated as two coefficients, which respectively represents real part and imaginary part (imaginary part only take coefficient)). Finally, the processed image is be retrieved by using the feature vector.

Table 1. Partial low intermediate frequency coefficient of encrypted medical image and variation after different attack.

Attack	Image manipulation	PSNR (dB)	ED(1,1)	ED(1,2)	ED(1,3)	ED(1,4)	ED(2,1)	ED(2,2)	ED(2,3)	ED(2,4)	symbolic sequence	NC
Conventional attack	Original encrypted image	90.275	146.69 +0.00i	-11.81- 0.42i	-17.54 -1.49i	-12.78 1.39i	-9.62 - 9.65i	-0.71 +1.06i	2.07 -0.99i	-0.53 +1.05i	11000000 10011001	1.0
	Gauss noise(1%)	20.375	148.39 +0.00i	-11.18 -0.32i	-17.24 -1.52i	-12.66 -1.40i	10.69 - 9.58i	-0.96 +0.91i	1.63 -1.11i	-0.66 +1.31i	11000000 10011001	1.0
	JPEG compression (10%)	18.488	4.45 +0.00i	-0.39- 0.02i	-0.62 -0.06i	-0.41- 0.05i	0.52 -0.40i	-0.02 +0.05i	0.04- 0.04i	-0.04 +0.05i	11000000 10011001	1.0
	Median filter [5x5]	21.623	143.06 + 0.00i	-13.04 - 1.11i	-18.19 -1.45i	-12.76 -1.01i	7.76 - 9.90i	-1.3 +0.97i	2.19 -0.47i	-0.36 +0.87i	11000000 10011001	1.0
Geometric attack	Clockwise rotation(5°)	16.345	145.86+ 0.00i	-12.16 + 0.11i	-17.08 - 1.40i	-12.85 -1.35i	7.92 - 9.36i	-0.01 + 0.67i	4.80- 0.70i	3.10 +0.98i	11010000 10011011	0.8
	Scaling(0.5)	--	36.67 +0.00i	-2.95 -0.18i	-4.36 -0.59i	-3.16- 0.58i	2.46 - 2.35i	-0.19 +0.26i	0.54- 0.21i	-0.16 +0.25i	11000000 10011001	1.0
	Left shift(5%)	15.950	144.1 +0.00i	-13.49 -4.69i	-15.03 -12.89i	-7.65 12.55i	-9.51 - 9.54i	-1.14 +0.86i	2.11 +0.64i	-1.31 +0.17i	11000000 10011101	0.9
	Down(5%)	14.250	145.0 +0.00i	-11.73 -0.36i	-17.45 -1.49i	-12.73- 1.36i	4.74 - 11.91i	-0.29 +1.28i	1.77 -1.55i	-0.16 +1.20i	11000000 10011001	1.0
	Y axis shear (5%)	--	145.0 +0.00i	-11.73 -0.36i	-17.45 -1.49i	-12.73 -1.36i	14.31 -11.55i	-1.42 +1.23i	1.10 -1.32i	-0.90 +1.20i	11000000 10011001	1.0

Notes:*2D-DFT transform coefficient unit 1.0e+005

By observing Table 1, we find that for conventional attack, the value of low intermediate frequency coefficients is almost constant. Although for geometric attacks, part of coefficient value has great change, it is easy to notice that although the majority of low intermediate frequency coefficient value has changed, its symbol has little changed.

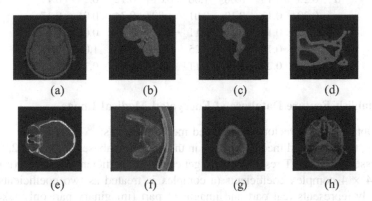

(a)   (b)   (c)   (d)

(e)   (f)   (g)   (h)

Fig. 2. Different original medical image, (a), (e), (g), (h) Head, (b)–(c) Liver, (d) shadow, (f) Teddy bear.

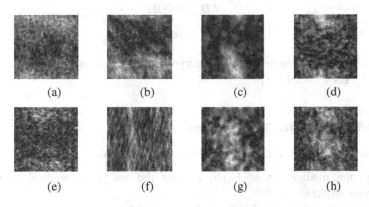

(a)   (b)   (c)   (d)

(e)   (f)   (g)   (h)

Fig. 3. Different encrypted medical image, (a), (e), (g), (h) Head, (b)–(c) Liver; (d) shadow, (f) Teddy bear.

We also encrypted different objects (shown in Fig. 2(a)–(h)) separately. And calculate the value of NC between each other (shown in Fig. 3), the result is shown in Table 2. From Table 2, we can find out that the value of NC between medical image itself is maximum, which is 1.00; it is not difficult to find that on two pieces of medical images, the more similar before encryption, the higher correlation coefficient of the extracted feature vector, which indicate the extracted feature vector reflects homomorphic characteristic of encrypted medical image.

Table 2. NC of different encryption medical image (length of vector is 32bit)

	a	b	c	d	e	f	g	h
a	1.00	0.38	0.19	−0.25	0.40	−0.12	0.00	0.64
b	0.38	1.00	0.31	−0.13	0.12	0.12	−0.12	0.27
c	0.19	0.31	1.00	−0.06	0.19	0.21	0.06	0.32
d	−0.25	−0.13	−0.06	1.00	−0.01	0.12	0.25	−0.12
e	0.39	0.11	0.19	−0.01	1.00	−0.34	0.01	0.17
f	−0.11	0.11	0.19	0.11	−0.32	1.00	0.02	−0.07
g	0.00	−0.12	0.06	0.25	0.01	0.02	1.00	0.12
h	0.62	0.26	0.31	−0.11	0.17	−0.07	0.11	1.00

3.3   Establish Feature Database of Encrypted Medical Image

Step 1. Obtain feature vector of encrypted medical images;

Firstly, the encrypted medical images in the image database E = {E1, E2, ⋯⋯, EN} are processed by 2D DFT respectively to get complex coefficient matrix ED(i, j). Then, the first 4 × 4 complex coefficients (a complex is treated as two coefficients, which respectively represents real part and imaginary part (imaginary part only take coefficient)) ED'(i, j) are selected to be computing by using threshold sign function SE(i) to obtain the feature vector of encrypted medical image EV(j).

$$SE(ED'(i,j)) = \begin{cases} 1 & ED'(i,j) \geq 0 \\ -1 & ED'(i,j) < 0 \end{cases} \quad (1 \leq i \leq 8, 1 \leq j \leq 4,) \qquad (5)$$

Step 2. Store the feature vector of encrypted medical images in feature database EV = {EV$_1$, EV$_2$, ⋯⋯, EV$_N$}.

3.4   Retrieve Encrypted Medical Image

Figure 4 is the model of encrypted medical image retrieval.

1. Encrypt the medical image F'(i, j) to gain the encrypted medical image E'(j) (Referring to 3.1);
2. Acquire the feature vector EV'(j) (Referring to 3.2);
3. Compute the NC between EV'(j) and EV(j);

    The Normalized Cross-correlation (NC) is used for measuring the quantitative similarity of two encrypted medical image, which is defined as:

$$NC = \frac{\sum_i \sum_j EV(j)EV'(j)}{\sum_i \sum_j EV^2(j)} \qquad (6)$$

4. Return the encrypted medical image on the basis of NC.

We can return the corresponding encrypted medical image with greatest NC value stored in image database.

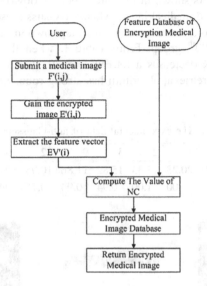

Fig. 4. The encrypted medical image retrieval model.

4 The Experimental Result

The simulation platform is MATLAB 2014a. In order to test and verify the correctness of assumptions about the algorithm mentioned above, we use 1000 groups of pseudo-random sequences only including 0 and 1. The length of every sequence is 32bit. We chose a groups from 1000 groups of pseudo-random sequence to put our target sequence (the 500th group was chosen in our experiment) extracted from a medical image randomly selected. We want to verify if our algorithm can retrieve the medical image under attacks. The medical image randomly-selected can be expressed as $F(i, j)$, in which $1 \leq i \leq 128$, $1 \leq j \leq 128$, and the corresponding DFT complex coefficient matrix is $FD(i, j)$; the encrypted medical image is expressed as $E(i, j)$, and the corresponding DFT coefficient matrix is $ED(i, j)$.

PSNR (Peak Signal to Noise Ratio) [14] is used to measure the distortion of the image. PSNR can be expressed as:

$$PSNR = 10 \lg \left[\frac{MN \max_{i,j}(I(i,j))^2}{\sum_i \sum_j (I(i,j) - \Gamma(i,j))^2} \right] \tag{7}$$

4.1   Interfered by Gaussian Noise

Add Gaussian noise into the encrypted medical image by using imnoise() function belonged to MATLAB. As shown in Fig. 5(a), there is obvious difference comparing with the original encrypted medical image when the Gauss noise intensity is 1%. Input this image into the detector, from the result which is shown in Fig. 5(b) the value of NC reach its peak in the 500th group. From Table 3, when the Gauss noise intensity increases to 18%, PSNR decreases a lot, NC = 0.79, it can still retrieve relatively, which indicates that the retrieval algorithm has strong robustness against the interference of Gaussian noise.

Table 3. The experimental data of anti-Gaussian noise

Noise (%)	1	2	3	9	12	15	18
PSNR (dB)	20.28	17.33	15.82	11.86	10.95	10.42	9.79
NC	1.00	1.00	0.94	0.94	0.76	0.87	0.79

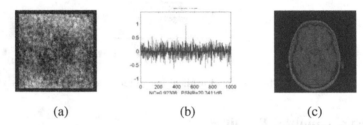

(a)   (b)   (c)

Fig. 5. Under Gaussian noise (1%) (a) the encrypted image, (b) the output of detector, (c) the decryption retrieved image.

4.2   JPEG Compressing Attack

JPEG compression procession is implemented by apply the percentage of image compression quality as a parameter. From Table 4, we can find when the compression percentage is only 10, the compression quality is low, NC = 0.83. Input an encrypted medical image (shown in Fig. 6(a)) into the detector, we can find from Fig. 6(b), the value of NC is at its peak in the 500th group, and the decryption retrieved image is shown in Fig. 6(c). From the results of the retrieval, we can get the conclusion that there is a good robustness against JPEG attack.

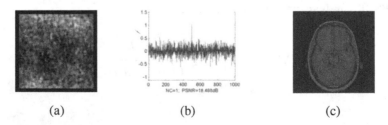

(a)   (b)   (c)

Fig. 6. Under JPEG compression attack (10%) (a) image under JPEG compression, (b) the output of detector, (c) the decryption retrieved image.

Table 4. The experimental data of anti JPEG compression

Percentage (%)	5	10	20	40	50	70	80
PSNR(dB)	17.98	18.07	18.25	18.31	18.32	18.31	18.32
NC	0.82	0.83	0.85	0.85	0.85	0.84	0.84

4.3 Median Filtering Attack

In this experiment, we change filtering window and filtering times separately to test the value of PSNR and NC of encrypted medical image, whose result is shown in Table 5. We find that its detail can't be seen after this image is filtered 10 times by using [5 × 5]. The processed image (shown in Fig. 7(a)) is used as the input of the detector, we can get the output result shown in Fig. 7(b) and the decryption retrieved image displayed in Fig. 7(c). The value of NC is at its peak in the 500th group, so we can hold that this encrypted algorithm has great robustness against median filtering attack.

Table 5. The experimental data of anti median filtering

	Median filter [3 × 3]			Median filter [5 × 5]			Median filter [7 × 7]		
Times	1	10	20	1	10	20	1	10	20
PSNR (dB)	28.70	25.01	24.94	24.66	21.62	21.34	22.38	20.49	19.59
NC	1.00	1.00	1.00	1.00	0.93	0.93	0.93	0.87	0.87

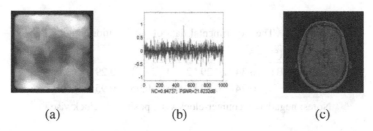

(a)	(b)	(c)

Fig. 7. Under median filtering attack [5 × 5] (10 times), (a) the encrypted image (b) the output result of detector (c) the decryption retrieved image.

4.4 Scaling Attack

We separately measure the value of NC, which represent zooming in and out, and the result is shown in Table 6. As we can see, when the scaling factor equal 0.5 (shown in Fig. 8(a)), NC = 0.93, add this image into the detector as input, and the output (shown in Fig. 8(b)). From the result of the detector, it is not hard to see the NC value of 500th group is the peak of all, and it prove that this algorithm has strong robustness against scaling attacks.

Table 6. The experimental data of anti scaling attack

Scaling	0.2	0.5	0.8	1.2	2	5	0.2	0.5
NC	0.72	0.93	0.93	1.00	1.00	1.00	0.72	0.93

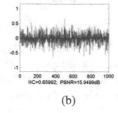

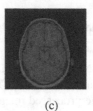

(a)   (b)   (c)

Fig. 8. Under scaling attack (0.5), (a) encrypted image, (b) the output result of detector, (c) the decryption retrieved image.

4.5 Rotation Attack

The value of PSNR and NC of the encrypted medical image after clockwise and counter-clockwise rotation is shown in Table 7. As seen from the table, when the encrypted image rotate clockwise with angle is 5° which is shown in Fig. 9(a), NC = 0.74. Input this image into detector, and get a responding display in Fig. 9(b), from which we can notice that the value of NC reach its peak in the 500th group. In conclusion, we can think that the algorithm has great robustness to rotation attack.

Table 7. The experimental data of anti rotation attack

Rotation (°)	−5	−2	−1	1	2	5
PSNR (dB)	16.34	20.29	24.61	24.61	20.29	16.35
NC	0.74	0.87	0.93	0.95	0.95	0.61

Notes: negative is counter-clockwise, positive is clockwise

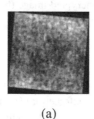

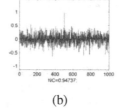

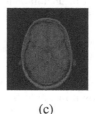

(a)   (b)   (c)

Fig. 9. Under rotation attack (5°), (a) encrypted image, (b) the output result of detector, (c) the decryption retrieved image.

4.6 Cropping Attack

The experimental data of the encrypted medical image resisting cropping attack is shown in Table 8, from which we can see that when 5% of the encrypted image is cut along Y axis, which is shown in Fig. 10(a), NC = 0.87. Add this image into the detector, and acquire the result (shown in Fig. 10(b)), from which it isn't difficult to find that the value of NC reach its peak in the 500th group. To sum up, this algorithm has strong robustness to against cropping attack.

Table 8. The experimental data of anti cropping attack

Percentage (%)	1	2	3	5	10
NC	1.00	1.00	0.87	0.87	0.74

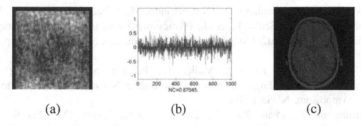

(a)	(b)	(c)

Fig. 10. Under cropping attack (5%), (a) the encrypted image, (b) the output result of detector, (c) the decryption retrieved image.

5 Conclusion

The experimental result prove that comparing with existing image retrieval algorithms based on content in plain text domain, the algorithm we proposed in this paper has strong robustness to resist Gauss noise and other conventional attacks, scaling, cropping and other geometric attacks. This algorithm can be able to quickly complete the retrieval operation.

Acknowledgement. This work is supported by the National Natural Science Foundation of China (No: 61263033), and by the International Science and Technology Cooperation Project of Hainan (No: KJHZ2015-04) and the Institutions of Higher Learning Scientific Research Special Project of Hainan Province (No: Hnkyzx2014-2).

References

1. Wang, Q., Megalooikonomou, V., Kontos, D.: Medical image retrieval framework. IEEE **28–30**, 233–238 (2005)
2. Shini, S.G., Thomas, T., Chithraranjan, K.: Cloud based medical image exchange security. Procedia Eng. **38**, 3454–3461 (2012)

3. Kokare, M., Chatterji, B.N., Biswas, P.K.: Cosine-modulated wavelet based texture features for content-based image retrieval. Pattern Recogn. Lett. **25**(4), 391–398 (2004)
4. Cheng, Q., Shen, Y., Shao, Z., Li, D.: Research on medical image retrieval based on arbitrary shape. In: IEEE, pp. 445–448 (2012)
5. Ng, V., Cheung, D., Fu, A.: Medical image retrieval by color content. In: IEEE, pp. 1980–1985 (1995)
6. Bellafqira, R., Coatrieux, G., Bouslimi, D., Quellec, G.: Content-based image retrieval in homomorphic encryption domain. In: IEEE, pp. 2944–2947 (2015)
7. Hrestak, D. Picek, S.: Homomorphic encryption in the cloud. In: IEEE, pp. 1400–1404 (2014)
8. Brenner, M., Perl, H., Smith, M.: How practical is homomorphically encrypted program execution? An implementation and performance evaluation. In: IEEE, pp. 375–382 (2012)
9. Erkin, Z., Franz, M., Guajardo, J., Katzenbeisser, S., Lagendijk, I., Toft, T.: Privacy-preserving face recognition. In: Goldberg, I., Atallah, Mikhail J. (eds.) PETS 2009. LNCS, vol. 5672, pp. 235–253. Springer, Heidelberg (2009). doi:10.1007/978-3-642-03168-7_14
10. Barni, M., Bianchi, T., Catalano, D., Di Raimondo, M., Labati, R.D., Failla, P., Fiore, D., Lazzeretti, R., Piuri, V., Scotti, F., et al.: Privacy-preserving fingercode authentication. In: Proceedings of the 12th ACM Workshop on Multimedia and Security, ACM, pp. 231–240 (2010)
11. Evans, D., Huang, Y., Katz, J., Malka, L.: Efficient privacy-preserving biometric identification. In: Proceedings of the 17th Conference Network and Distributed System Security Symposium, NDSS (2011)
12. Rahulamathavan, Y., Phan, R.C.-W., Chambers, J.A., Parish, D.J.: Facial expression recognition in the encrypted domain based on local fisher discriminant analysis. IEEE Trans. Affect. Compute **4**(1), 83–92 (2013)
13. Wu, J., Wang, X., Yan, D., Wei, C., Zhang, Y.: Method for medical image retrieval based on frequency layer feature. IEEE, vol 2, pp. 622–624 (2009)
14. Tanchenko, A.: Visual-PSNR measure of image quality. J. Vis. Commun. Image Represent. **25**, 874–878 (2014)

A Robust Watermarking Algorithm
for Medical Images in the Encrypted Domain

Jiangtao Dong, Jingbing Li[⊠], and Zhen Guo

College of Information Science and Technology,
Hainan University, Haikou, China
jingbingli2008@hotmail.com

Abstract. Most of the existing robust watermarking schemes were designed to embed the watermark information into the plaintext images, which leads to a latent risk of exposing information and are vulnerable to unauthorized access. In addition, the robustness of watermarking in the encrypted domain is another issue that should be taken into account. Based on Discrete Fourier Transform (DFT) and Logistic chaotic map, we proposed a robust zero-watermarking algorithm in the DFT encrypted domain, which achieves good safety in the protection of both watermark information and the original image itself. Firstly, we encrypt the watermark and the original medical image in DFT encrypted domain. Then, the DFT is performed on the encrypted medical image to acquire the feature vector. In watermark embedding and extraction phase, zero-watermarking technique is utilized to ensure integrity of medical image. Experimental results demonstrate good robustness against both common attacks and geometric distortions.

Keywords: Robustness · Encrypted domain · DFT · Logistic chaotic map · Zero-watermarking

1 Introduction

With the rapid advance of network technology, multimedia information can easily been accessed by unauthorized person. Digital watermarking is a technique that has been developed for protecting digital information. However, the security of watermarking is a challenging issue in watermarking community. For most existing watermarking schemes, the embedding and extraction phases are performed on the plaintext images [1], which leads to a latent risk of exposing information. Thus, to process in the encrypted domain is a reasonable solution to this problem. There are many robust watermarking schemes in the plaintext domain, such as in [2, 3], which achieved good robustness under both common attacks and geometric distortions. However, transplanting these existing watermarking schemes directly to the encrypted domain is a complicated work, due to the limitation of the encryption. The robustness of the watermark in the encrypted domain is another issue that should be taken into account [1].

In 1978, Rivest, Adleman and Derouzos published a paper of homomorphic encryption [4]. The homomorphic cryptosystems provide a suitable way for signal processing in the encrypted domain, since they retain the algebraic relations between the plaintext and the encrypted image. Since then, several homomorphic cryptosystems

© Springer International Publishing AG 2017
C. Xing et al. (Eds.): ICSH 2016, LNCS 10219, pp. 217–229, 2017.
DOI: 10.1007/978-3-319-59858-1_21

have been proposed. Among them, the fully homomorphic cryptosystems allow the computation of any polynomial in the encrypted domain [5]. Gentry's fully homomorphic encryption scheme [6] is a great theoretical breakthrough of the homomorphic cryptosystems. Over the past few years, numerous works on signal processing in the encrypted domain had been reported. The implementations of the Discrete Fourier Transform (DFT) and the Fast Fourier Transform (FFT) in the encrypted domain were proposed by Bianchi et al. [7]. They also conducted an investigation in the encrypted DCT domain [8]. Zheng et al. proposed the implementation of DWT in the encrypted domain [9]. And other processing includes composite signal representation [10], privacy-preserving face recognition [11], image feature extraction in the encrypted domain with privacy-preserving scale-invariant feature transform (SIFT) [12], and a recommendation system in the encrypted domain [13]. A Walsh-Hadamard transform based image watermarking scheme in the encrypted domain was proposed by Zheng et al. [14] in which the embedding and extraction processes could be performed by a third party without leaking images.

In this paper, we proposed a robust watermarking algorithm in the encrypted domain. In Sect. 3, we proposed a zero-watermarking scheme in the DFT encrypted domain. In Sect. 4, through the experimental results we discussed the robustness of our algorithm under various kinds of attacks. We concluded our paper in Sect. 5.

2 The Fundamental Theory

2.1 The Discrete Fourier Transform (DFT)

The Discrete Fourier Transform is a signal analysis theory. The M × N medical image's DFT is done using:

$$F(u,v) = \sum_{x=0}^{M-1} \sum_{y=0}^{N-1} f(x,y) \cdot e^{-j2\pi xu/M} e^{-j2\pi yv/N}$$

$$u = 0, 1, \ldots, M-1 \; ; \; v = 0, 1, \ldots, N-1$$

(1)

The M × N medical image's Inverse Discrete Fourier Transform (IDFT) is defined by:

$$f(x,y) = \frac{1}{MN} \sum_{u=0}^{M-1} \sum_{v=0}^{N-1} F(u,v) e^{j2\pi \left(\frac{ux}{M} + \frac{vy}{N} \right)}$$

$$x = 0, 1, \ldots, M-1 \; ; \; y = 0, 1, \ldots, N-1$$

(2)

where f(x, y) corresponds to the value of the medical image at point (x, y) and F(u, v) matches the DFT coefficient at point (u, v) in frequency domain. Digital images are usually expressed in pixels square, so we set M = N.

2.2 Logistic Map

A chaotic system has a noise like behavior while it is exactly deterministic so we can reproduce it if we have its parameters and initial values. These signals are extremely sensitive to initial conditions [15]. One of the most famous chaotic systems is Logistic Map, which is a nonlinear return map given by

$$x_{k+1} = x_k(1 - x_k) \tag{3}$$

Where $0 \leq \mu \leq 4$ and $x_k \in (0,1)$ are the system variable and parameter respectively, and k is the number of iteration. Logistic Map system works under chaotic condition when $3.569945 \leq \mu \leq 4$. It can be seen that a small difference in initial conditions would lead to a significant difference of chaotic sequences. These statistical characteristics are the same as white noise, so the above sequence is an ideal secret-key sequence. In this paper, we set $\mu = 4$, and the chaotic sequences are generated by different initial values.

3 The Fundamental Theory

3.1 Encryption Algorithm of the Original Medical Images and Watermark Images

Step 1. Encryption of the medical images.

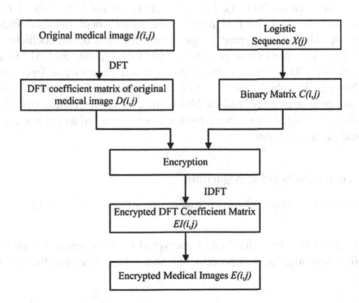

Fig. 1. Encryption of original medical images

Figure 1 is the flow chart of encrypting the original medical image. The encryption procedures are as follows:

(1) acquiring the DFT coefficients $D(i, j)$ by using the Discrete Fourier Transform;
(2) using Logistic Map to achieve the chaotic sequence $X(j)$, then we can get the binary matrix $C(i, j)$ by sign operation and dimension raising process;
(3) utilizing dot multiplication algorithm to process $D(i, j)$ and $C(i, j)$ to acquire the encrypted DFT coefficient matrix $EI(i, j)$;
(4) implementing inverse Discrete Fourier Transform (IDFT) for $EI (i, j)$ to obtain the encrypted medical image $E(i, j)$.

$$D(i,j) = \text{DFT2}(I(i,j)) \tag{4}$$

$$EI(i,j) = D(i,j) . * C(i,j) \tag{5}$$

$$E(i,j) = \text{IDFT2} (EI(i,j)) \tag{6}$$

Step 2. Encryption of the watermark images.

Using the similar approach as encrypting the original medical images to encrypt the original watermark images.

3.2 Acquire the Feature Vector of Encrypted Medical Images

Firstly, the original encrypted image is computed by using DFT. Then, we choose 5 low-frequency coefficients (F(1, 1), F(1, 2), ...F(1, 5)) for formation of the feature vector, as shown in Table 1. We find that the value of the low-frequent coefficients may change after attacking the encrypted image, while the signs of the coefficients remain unchanged. Let "1" represents a positive or zero coefficient, and "0" represents a negative coefficient. Then we can obtain the sign sequence of low-frequency coefficients, as shown in the column "Sequence of coefficient signs" in Table 1. After attack, the sign sequence is unchanged, and the Normalized Cross-correlation (NC) is equal to 1.0. This means that the signs of the sequence can be regarded as the feature vector of the encrypted medical images.

3.3 Watermark Embedding Algorithm

Figure 2 is the flow chart of embedding watermark images. The embedding procedures are as follows:

(1) Acquiring the feature vector $V(j)$ of encrypted medical images by using DFT;
(2) Applying hash algorithm to process $V(j)$ and $EW(j)$ to acquire the key sequence $Key(j)$;

$$FD(i,j) = DFT2(E(i,j)) \qquad (7)$$

$$V(j) = sign(FD(i,j)) \qquad (8)$$

$$Key(j) = V(j) \oplus EW(j) \qquad (9)$$

Table 1. Change of DFT coefficients under different attacks to encrypted medical images

Image processing	PSNR (dB)	F(1,1)	F(1,2)	F(1,3)	F(1,4)	F(1,5)	Sequence of coefficient signs	NC
Encrypted original image	-	9.20+0i	0.88+2.90i	-0.72-0.43i	-0.92-0.35i	-0.25-0.26i	1001000000	1.00
Gaussian noise (1%)	20.89	9.53+0i	0.80+2.77i	-0.70-0.43i	-0.86-0.31i	-0.23-0.25i	1001000000	1.00
JPEG compression (10%)	20.25	5.87+0i	0.63+2.20i	-0.60-0.33i	-0.58-0.28i	-0.09-0.22i	1001000000	1.00
Median filter [5x5](20 times)	25.25	8.94+0i	0.90+2.98i	-0.71-0.44i	-0.94-0.35i	-0.27-0.25i	1001000000	1.00
Rotation (clockwise, 5°)	17.95	9.14+0i	0.87+2.91i	-0.75-0.37i	-0.87-0.31i	-0.22-0.14i	1001000000	1.00
Scaling(×0.5)	-	2.30+0i	0.23+0.71i	-0.17-0.11i	-0.22-0.10i	-0.05-0.07i	1001000000	1.00
Translation(5%, left)	17.79	9.15+0i	1.48+2.66i	-0.55-0.69i	-0.61-0.82i	-0.03-0.39i	1001000000	1.00
Cropping(10%,Y direction)	-	8.45+0i	0.82+2.68i	-0.70-0.38i	-0.82-0.32i	-0.25-0.27i	1001000000	1.00

DFT transform coefficient unit: 1.0e+005

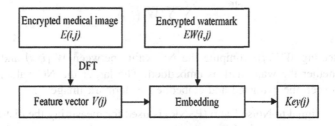

Fig. 2. Watermark embedding algorithm.

3.4 Watermark Extraction Algorithm

Figure 3 is the flow chart of extracting watermark image. The extraction procedures are as follows:

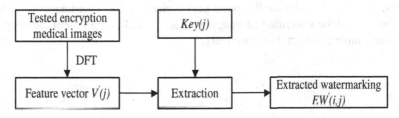

Fig. 3. Watermark extraction algorithm

(1) Acquire the feature vector $V'(j)$ of the tested encrypted medical images by using the Discrete Fourier Transform (DFT) and sign operation;

(2) Applying hash algorithm to process $V'(j)$ and Key (j) to acquire the encryption watermark sequence $EW'(j)$;

$$FD'(i,j) = \text{DFT2}(E'(i,j)) \tag{10}$$

$$V'(j) = \text{sign}(FD'(i,j)) \tag{11}$$

$$EW'(j) = Key(j) \oplus V'(j) \tag{12}$$

3.5   Watermark Evaluation Algorithm

(1) The Normalized Cross-correlation (NC) is used for measuring the quantitative similarity between the embedded and extracted original watermark, which is defined as:

$$NC = \frac{\sum_i \sum_j W(i,j)W'(i,j)}{\sum_i \sum_j W^2(i,j)} \tag{13}$$

After detecting $W'(i,j)$, compute the NC value between W (i, j) and $W'(i,j)$ to determine whether the watermark is embedded. The larger the NC value, the higher similarity between the extracted and embedded watermark image is.

(2) The Peak Signal to Noise Ratio (PSNR) is used for measuring the distortion of the watermarked image, which is defined as:

$$PSNR = 10\lg \left[\frac{MN \max_{i,j}(I(i,j))^2}{\sum_i \sum_j (I(i,j) - I'(i,j))^2} \right] \tag{14}$$

where $I(i, j)$ and $I'(i, j)$ denote the pixel gray values of the coordinates (i, j) in the original image and the watermarked images respectively; M, N represent the image row and column numbers of pixels respectively.

4   Experiments and Results

In our experiment, we select the tenth slice of one medical volume medical data as the original medical image and choose a significant binary image as the original watermark image. Figure 4(a) shows the original medical image. Figure 5(a) shows the original binary image $W = \{W(i, j) \mid W(i, j) = 0, 1; 1 \leq i \leq 32, 1 \leq j \leq 32\}$. The parameters for encrypting the binary watermark images are: $x_0 = 0.2$, $\mu = 4$; and the parameters for encrypting the medical images are: $x_0' = 0.135, \mu' = 4$.

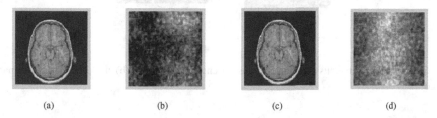

Fig. 4. Encryption and decryption of medical image: (a) original medical images, (b) the encrypted image, (c) decrypted image using the right key, (d) decrypted image using a wrong key

Fig. 5. Encryption and decryption of binary watermark image: (a) original watermark image, (b) the scrambled watermark image, (c) decrypted watermark image using the right key, (d) decrypted watermark image using a wrong key.

Figure 4(b)–(d) are the encrypted medical image, the decrypted image using the right key, and the decrypted image using a wrong key respectively. Figure 5(b)–(d) are the encrypted medical image, the decrypted image using the right key, and the decrypted image using a wrong key respectively. The safety of the proposed algorithm depends on the sensitiveness of the initial value of Logistic chaotic sequence.

To verify the effectiveness of the proposed algorithm, we carried out the simulation on Matlab R2010a platform to test the robustness of withstanding common attacks and geometric attacks.

4.1 Common Attacks

1. Gaussian noise attacks

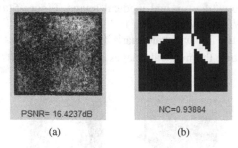

(a)   (b)

Fig. 6. Images under Gaussian noise (3%): (a) encrypted image, (b) the extracted watermark image

Table 2. The PSNR and NC under gaussian noise attack

Noise (%)	1	3	5	10	15	20	25
PSNR(dB)	20.84	16.43	14.53	12.06	10.62	9.81	9.20
NC	0.96	0.93	0.84	0.82	0.78	0.81	0.82

Figure 6(a) shows the medical image under Gaussian noise (3%) attacks with PSNR = 16.4237 dB. The similarity can be detected with NC = 0.9388, as shown in Fig. 6(b). Table 2 shows the NC values between the extracted and embedded watermark, and the PSNR values of the attacked encryption medical image. The data proved that our proposed algorithm has strong robustness against Gaussian noise attacks.

2. JPEG compression attacks

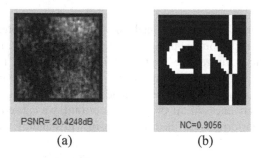

(a)   (b)

Fig. 7. Images under JPEG compression (20%): (a) encrypted image, (b) the extracted watermark image

Table 3. The PSNR and NC under JPEG compression

JPEG factor (%)	2	4	8	10	20	40	60	80
PSNR (dB)	20.10	20.13	20.19	20.25	20.42	20.52	20.60	20.65
NC	0.90	0.84	0.84	0.84	0.90	0.90	0.90	0.90

JPEG compression is done by using the of image quality percentage as a parameter. The watermarked image with PSNR = 20.4248 dB under JPEG attacks (20%) is shown in Fig. 7(a). The watermark can be extracted with NC = 0.9056, as shown in Fig. 7(b). Table 3 gives the PSNR and NC values for watermark extraction under different JPEG compression quality. Results show that the watermarking algorithm has strong robustness against JPEG compression attacks.

3. Median filtering attacks

We also explore the filter impact on the watermarked medical image with different size of median filters and filtering numbers. The watermarked image with PSNR= 29.5538 dB under median filtering [3 × 3] (1 time) is shown in Fig. 8(a). As shown in Fig. 8(b), the extracted watermark can obviously be seen with NC = 1.00. Table 4 gives the PSNR and NC values for watermark extraction under different median filter parameters. Results show that the watermarking algorithm has strong robustness against median filtering attacks.

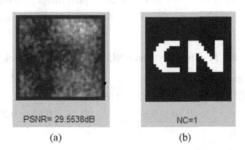

(a)   (b)

Fig. 8. Images under median filtering [3 × 3] (1time): (a) encrypted image, (b) the extracted watermark image

Table 4. The PSNR and NC under median filtering

	Median filter [3 × 3]			Median filter [5 × 5]			Median filter [7 × 7]		
Filtering times	1	10	20	1	10	20	1	10	20
PSNR (dB)	29.55	25.56	25.50	25.25	22.14	21.84	23.36	21.05	20.17
NC	1.00	0.90	0.90	1.00	0.96	0.96	1.00	0.83	0.69

4.2   Geometrical Attacks

1. Rotation attack.

We investigate the effectiveness of our proposed watermarking algorithm against rotation attacks with rotation angle as parameter. The medical image under 2°, clockwise rotation attacks, which has PSNR value of 21.5776 dB, as shown in Fig. 9. And the extracted watermark can be detected with NC = 0.84444. Table 5 gives the PSNR values of the attacked watermarked image, which proves that the proposed algorithm has strong robustness against rotation attacks.

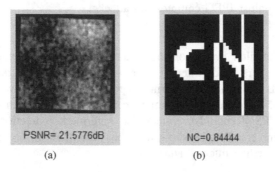

| | (a) | (b) |

Fig. 9. Images under rotation (2°, clockwise): (a) encrypted image, (b) the extracted watermark image

Table 5. The PSNR and NC under rotation attack

Rotation (°)	−1	−2	−3	−4	−5	−10
PSNR (dB)	25.79	21.57	19.69	18.61	17.95	16.33
NC	0.90	0.84	0.75	0.71	0.65	0.52

2. Scaling attacks

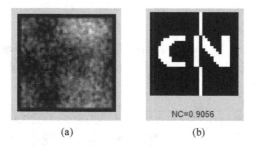

| | (a) | (b) |

Fig. 10. Images under scaling (0.5 times): (a) encrypted image, (b) the extracted watermark image

We utilize scaling factor as parameters to validate the effectiveness of our proposed algorithm on different scaling attacks. Figure 10(a) shows a watermarked image shrunk with a scale factor of 0.5. Figure 10(b) shows that the corresponding watermark can be extracted with NC = 0.9056. Table 6 shows the NC values between the embedded and extracted watermarking with scaling attacks on the watermarked images with multiple scale parameters, which can prove that our proposed algorithm has strong robustness against scaling attacks.

Table 6. The PSNR and NC under scaling attack

Scaling	0.2	0.5	0.8	1	1.2	2	4	6
NC	0.67	0.90	0.90	1.00	1.00	1.00	1.00	0.96

3. Translation attacks

The translation attacks are added to the watermarked image for validating the effectiveness of our proposed algorithm. Figure 11 shows an encrypted medical image translated by 1% vertical translation, downwardly, which achieves PSNR value of 24.1747 dB. Moreover, as shown in Fig. 11(b), the watermark can be detected with NC = 1.00. Table 7 gives the PSNR values of the attacked watermark image and the NC values between the embedded and extracted watermarking after translation attacks, which can prove that our algorithm has strong robustness against translation attacks.

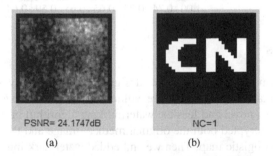

PSNR= 24.1747dB   NC=1

(a)   (b)

Fig. 11. Images under translation (1%, down): (a) encrypted image, (b) the extracted watermark image

Table 7. The PSNR and NC under translation

Percent (%)	1	2	4	6	8	10
PSNR (dB)	24.17	19.96	16.79	16.07	15.34	14.87
NC	1	0.80	0.80	0.76	0.54	0.49

4. Cropping attacks

The cropping attacks are added to the watermarked image for validating the effectiveness of our proposed algorithm. Figure 12 shows that the medical image cropping from Y direction, 2%. Moreover, Fig. 12(b) shows that watermark with NC = 0.74565 can be detected. Table 8 gives the NC values between the embedded and extracted watermarking with cropping attacks on the watermarked images, which can prove that our proposed algorithm has strong robustness against cropping attacks.

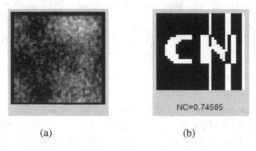

(a)   (b)

Fig. 12. Images under cropping (2%, Y direction): (a) encrypted image, (b) the extracted watermark image

Table 8. The PSNR and NC under cropping attack (from Y direction)

Cropping ratio (%)	1	2	4	6	8	10	20	30
NC	1.00	0.74	0.74	0.65	0.65	0.59	0.64	0.50

5   Conclusions

The existing watermarking schemes were designed to embed the watermark information into the original images, which are vulnerable to unauthorized access. In this paper, we proposed a novel and feasible watermarking algorithm in the DFT encrypted domain. First, we encrypted both the original medical image and the watermark image by using DFT and Logistic map; Then we embedded watermark into encrypted image. In watermarking embedding and extraction phase, zero-watermarking technique was utilized to ensure the integrity of medical images. At the end of the paper, we compared the robustness of watermarking algorithm between the unencrypted and encrypted approach. Results demonstrate that the watermarking approach in the encrypted domain obtains not only good robustness against common attacks and geometric attacks, but also ideal homomorphism, which can be utilized in the protection of both original image and watermark image.

Acknowledgments. This research was supported by National Natural Science Foundation of China (NO. 61263033), and by International Science and Technology Cooperation Project of Hainan (NO. KJHZ2015-04) and the Institutions of Higher Learning Scientific Research Special Project of Hainan (NO. Hnkyzx2014-2), and Natural Science Foundation of Hainan (NO. 20166217).

References

1. Guo, J., Zheng, P., Huang, J.: Secure watermarking scheme against watermark attacks in the encrypted domain. J. Vis. Commun. Image R. **30**, 125–135 (2015)
2. Deng, C., Gao, X., Li, X., Tao, D.: A local tchebichef moments-based robust image watermarking. Sig. Process. **89**(8), 1531–1539 (2009)
3. Gao, X., Deng, C., Li, X., Tao, D.: Geometric distortion insensitive image watermarking in affine covariant regions. IEEE Trans. Syst. Man Cybernet. Part C: Appl. Rev. **40**(3), 278–286 (2010)
4. Rivest, R.L., Adleman, L., Dertouzos, M.L.: On data banks and privacy homomorphisms. Found. Secure Comput. **4**(11), 169–180 (1978)
5. Aguilar-Melchor, C., Fau, S., Fontaine, C., Gogniat, G., Sirdey, R.: Recent advances in homomorphic encryption: a possible future for signal processing in the encrypted domain. IEEE Signal Process. Mag. **30**, 108–117 (2013)
6. Gentry, C.: Fully homomorphic encryption using ideal lattices. In: Proceedings of the Forty-first Annual ACM Symposium on Theory of Computing, ACM, pp. 169–178 (2009)
7. Bianchi, T., Piva, A., Barni, M.: On the implementation of the discrete fourier transform in the encrypted domain. IEEE Trans. Inform. Forensics Secur. **4**(1), 86–97 (2009)
8. Bianchi, T., Piva, A., Barni, M.: Encrypted domain DCT based on homomorphic cryptosystems. EURASIP J. Inform., Secur (2009)
9. Zheng, P., Huang, J.: Discrete wavelet transform and data expansion reduction in homomorphic encrypted domain. IEEE Trans. Image Process. **22**, 2455–2468 (2013)
10. Bianchi, T., Piva, A., Barni, M.: Composite signal representation for fast and storage-efficient processing of encrypted signals. IEEE Trans. Inform. Forensics Secur. **5**(1), 180–187 (2010)
11. Erkin, Z., Franz, M., Guajardo, J., Katzenbeisser, S., Lagendijk, I., Toft, T.: Privacy-preserving face recognition. In: Goldberg, I., Atallah, Mikhail J. (eds.) PETS 2009. LNCS, vol. 5672, pp. 235–253. Springer, Heidelberg (2009). doi:10.1007/978-3-642-03168-7_14
12. Hsu, C.-Y., Lu, C.-S., Pei, S.-C.: Image feature extraction in encrypted domain with privacy-preserving sift. IEEE Trans. Image Process. **21**, 4593–4607 (2012)
13. Shieh, J.-R., Lin, C.-Y., Wu, J.-L.: Recommendation in the end-to-end encrypted domain. In: Proceedings of the 20th ACM International Conference on Information and Knowledge Management, ACM, pp. 915–924 (2011)
14. Zheng, P., Huang, J.: Walsh-hadamard transform in the homomorphic encrypted domain and its application in image watermarking. In: Kirchner, M., Ghosal, D. (eds.) IH 2012. LNCS, vol. 7692, pp. 240–254. Springer, Heidelberg (2013). doi:10.1007/978-3-642-36373-3_16
15. Sabery, M., Yaghoobi, K.M.: A new approach for image encryption using chaotic logistic map. In: Proceedings of 2008 International Conference of the IEEE on Advanced Computer Theory and Engineering, pp. 585–590 (2008)

Effect of a Mobile Internet Regional Cooperative Rescue System on Reperfusion Efficiency and Prognosis of STEMI Patients

Sijun Yu[1], Yu Yang[2(✉)], Wei Han[1(✉)], Jing Lu[1(✉)], and Huiliang Liu[1(✉)]

[1] Department of Cardiology, General Hospital of Chinese People's Armed Police Forces, Beijing, China
rdysj@163.com, cardiology2007@sina.com, lujj1016@icloud.com, lh1518@vip.sina.com
[2] Department of Medical Affairs, General Hospital of Chinese People's Armed Police Forces, Beijing, China
yysbox@126.com

Abstract. **Objective:** To explore the effect of a mobile Internet regional cooperative rescue system on reperfusion efficiency and prognosis of patients with ST segment elevation myocardial infarction (STEMI). **Methods:** The patients were divided into two groups: the regional transported group (experimental group) and routine transported group (control group) according to whether the first medical contact (FMC) unit was equipped with a regional cooperative rescue system. Every time point during transport process, the time to peak and peak value of cardiac troponin I (cTNI), the rate of heart failure or cardiac death during hospitalization, the value of ejection fractions (EF) measured in 24 h, and indicators of health economics(total hospital charges, days) were observed. **Results:** The difference of time delay between two groups were all statistically significant $P(<0.05)$; the peak time of cTnI was earlier in experimental group than control group ((14.2 ± 3.4) h vs. (16.3 ± 4.6) h, $P < 0.01$), the peak value of cTnI was decreased in experimental group compared with the control group ((9.3 ± 2.9) ng/ml vs. (12.3 ± 3.2) ng/ml, $P < 0.01$); values of EF within 24 h after admission were significantly lower in control group than experimental group ($t = 2.37$, $P < 0.05$); in-hospital heart failure rate of experimental group was less than that of the control group $2\chi(= 4.46, P = 0.03)$; cardiac mortality rate of experimental group was less than that of the control group, and it was not significant between the two groups ($\chi 2 = 0.19$, $P = 0.66$); total cost in hospital, total hospital stay were significantly decreased in experimental group compared with the control group ((56711 ± 12083) yuan vs. (65847 ± 14691) yuan, $P < 0.01$; (6.35 ± 3.68)d vs. the day (8.64 ± 5.19)d, $P = 0.01$). **Conclusions:** Regional cooperative rescue system could significantly shorten the time delay of patients with STEMI, improve heart function in acute stage and reduce the time and cost in hospital.

Keywords: Regional cooperative rescue system · ST-segment elevation myocardial infarction · First medical contact to device time · Door-to-balloon time

© Springer International Publishing AG 2017
C. Xing et al. (Eds.): ICSH 2016, LNCS 10219, pp. 230–237, 2017.
DOI: 10.1007/978-3-319-59858-1_22

1   Introduction

Along with the development of social economic, the incidence of acute myocardial infarction (AMI) showed a trend of rising year by year. Statistics show that cardiovascular disease has already become the chief cause of death in China, and myocardial infarction is a critical emergency situation [1]. Large-scale clinical studies have confirmed that every 30 min delay lead to 7.5% rise in myocardial infarction mortality rate in 1 year [2], while restoration of infarction related vascular blood flow timely can improve prognosis and reduce mortality. Qin divided the total time delay into four parts: the patient's delay, emergency medical system, transport delay, and hospital delay [3]. In 2013 the American Heart Association (AHA) recommended the first medical contact to device time (FMC-D) as an index to evaluate the efficacy of acute ST segment elevation myocardial infarction (STEMI) treatment for the first time. FMC-D refers to the duration from when the first medical unit (regardless of the level and category) reached STEMI patients to when the coronary blood flow reserved by interventional devices [4]. At present, China's delay in treatment of myocardial infarction consists of the patient's own delay (60%), emergency medical system delay (10%), transport delay (10%), hospital delays (20%). That is, FMC-D time accounted for 40% of the total delay. At the present stage most of the domestic regions still committed to build the green channel to shorten 20% of hospital delays. Some advanced regions are trying to establish regional coordination treatment system with emergency medical service (EMS) and the PCI medical institutions, in order to shorten the 40% delay within medical system. The author's hospital has established a Regional Cooperative Rescue System (RCRS) including PCI capable hospitals and non-PCI capable medical units (including community clinics, hospitals and EMS) based of mobile communication and information technology. In this study we try to evaluate effect of this system on STEMI treatment in the author's hospital.

2   Objective and Methods

2.1   Objective

Patients diagnosed as STEMI from General Hospital of Chinese People's Armed Police Forces (GHCAPF) during 12/2014 to 6/2015 were continuously enrolled in our study. All of them were scheduled for Primary Percutaneous Coronary Intervention (PPCI). They were divided into two groups: the regional transported group (experimental group) and the routine transported group (control group) according to whether the first medical contact (FMC) unit was equipped with a regional cooperative rescue system terminal. STEMI was diagnosed as: (1) typical symptoms persist for more than 30 min, which-cannot alleviate after the application of nitrates. (2) Elevation of ST segment in 2 or more than 2 adjacent leads in any of the following conditions: male $\geq$0.2 mV, female $\geq$0.1 mV (V2–V3), while in other chest leads or limb leads $\geq$0.1 mV; Existence of Q wave. (3) The myocardial enzymes such as creatine kinase isoenzyme (CK-MB), or troponin T or I increased [5]. Heart failure was diagnosed according to the Killip classification standard [6]. The Killip heart function after myocardial infarction in Class 2 or 2 above is defined as heart failure.

2.2 Methods

Treatment. All patients were given aspirin 300 mg and Plavix 600 mg chewing immediately after the diagnosis was made. They were transported to GHCAPF in two different ways and underwent PPCI unless contraindicated. All of patients were given conventional angiotensin converting enzyme inhibitors, beta-blockers, statins, aspirin, Plavix and other drugs if necessary after the procedure.

Regional Cooperative Rescue System (RCRS). With the comprehensive utilization of information engineering, mobile communication and clinical medicine, we build a STEMI treatment information platform. We use this platform to build a regional collaborative rescue system, which made the emergency medical system (EMS), non-PCI capable medical units and PCI capable hospitals in a certain region as a whole rescue system for STEMI. When the patient reached the FMC medical unit with an RCRS terminal, he was enrolled in the RCRS system. We use a cloud computing system to calculate which is the "nearest" (most efficient rescue efficacy for this very patient if more precisely) surrounding PCI capable hospital. And a message including 12 or 18 leads ECG, other vital signs and geographic information were transferred to a cardiologist in this "nearest" hospital. If the diagnosis of STEMI was made and PPCI was indicated, the patient was directly transported to this hospital's cathlab as soon as possible. For emergency surgery, EMS terminal through the GPRS satellite positioning system and mobile base station signal generation and positioning, and positioning based on the location of the server to be sent to the location of the calculation. The cloud computing server use LBS cloud technology, cloud retrieval based on terminal position information and hospital distribution, ant colony algorithm, neural network algorithm, particle swarm algorithm and path planning algorithm to calculate the best transport route to avoid the real-time traffic congestion. At the same time, the cloud computing server use the medical data (D-B time and survival rate) of the surrounding hospitals for big data analysis. Based on the above geographic data and medical results, the server gives the optimal destined hospital and informed the interventional cardiologists to be prepared for PPCI (Figs. 1 and 2).

Routine Treatment of STEMI. The patient was transported to or self-arrived at the emergency department of our hospital. ED called for cardiologist's consultation if STEMI was suspicious. The cardiologist confirmed the diagnosis of STEMI based on ECG and other medical data and transferred the patient to cathlab for PPCI if indicated (Fig. 3).

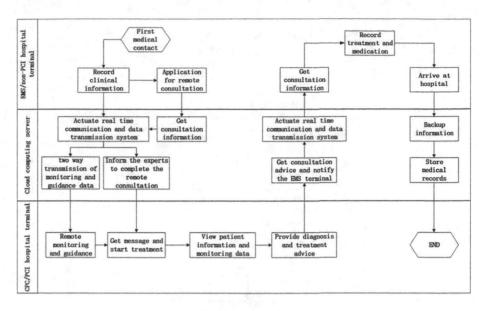

Fig. 1. Algorithm of RCRS

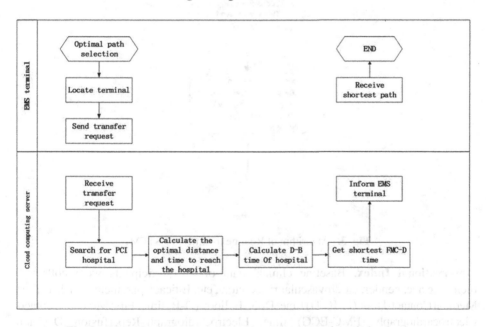

Fig. 2. Algorithm of communication between terminals and cloud server

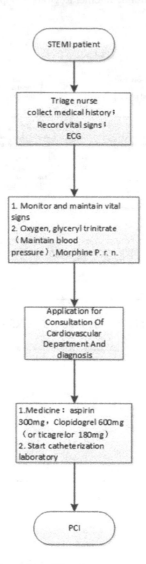

Fig. 3. Algorithm of Routine treatment of STEMI

Observational Index. Baseline clinical data of the participants were collected, including age, gender, cardiovascular risk factors, etc. Efficacy parameters such as First Medical Contact-Door (FMC-D) time, Door-Balloon (D-B) time, First Medical Contact-Electrocardiograph (FMC-ECG) time, Electrocardiograph–Reperfusion Decision (ECG-Reperfusion Decision) time were also calculated. Cardiac Troponin I (cTnI) in 2 h, 8 h, 16 h, 24 h, 48 h after PPCI was checked to find out the peak value and peak time of cTnI. The incidence of in-hospital heart failure and mortality were also compare in two groups. 24 h EF after operation was also recorded. Health economic parameters such as total hospital stay and cost were also analyzed.

3   Results

3.1   Baseline Data

57 patients were included in the experimental group, with 32 male, 25 female, average ages 63.2 ± 11.6 years old. 61 were enrolled in the control group, with 36 male, 25 female, average ages 62.4 ± 13.5 years old. All of the above showed no statistically significant differences (P > 0.05). Risk factors such as hypertension, diabetes, overweight, smoking, alcohol, and hyperlipidemia had no differences between two groups (P > 0.05).

3.2   Efficiency Parameters

There are statistically differences between efficiency parameters of two groups; comparison of FMC-D time [(113.5 ± 32.7) min vs. (135.6 ± 57.2) min, P < 0.05], comparison of D-B time [(61.3 ± 27.4) min vs. (79.3 ± 28.6) min, P < 0.05], comparison of cases and rate that meet the FMC-D time standard (FMC-D≤120 min) [35 (61.4) vs. 26 (42.6), P < 0.05], comparison of cases and rate that meet D-B time standard (D-B ≤ 90 min) [53 (93.0) vs. 48 (78.7), P < 0.05], comparison of FMC-ECG time [(2.4 ± 0.6) min vs. (4.3 ± 1.7) min, P < 0.05], comparison of ECG-Reperfusion Decision time [(23.2 ± 7.1) min vs. (61.7 ± 23.1) min, P < 0.05] (Table 1).

Table 1. Efficiency Parameters

Group	FMC-D (min)	D-B (min)	FMC-ECG (min)	ECG-D (min)	D-B ≤ 90 min [n (%)]	FMC-D ≤ 120 min [n (%)]
experimental group ($n = 57$)	113.5 ± 32.7	61.3 ± 27.4	2.4 ± 0.6	23.2 ± 7.1	53 (93.0)	35 (61.4)
Control group ($n = 61$)	135.6 ± 57.2	79.3 ± 28.6	4.3 ± 1.7	61.7 ± 23.1	48 (78.7)	26 (42.6)
χ^2/t	−2.55	−3.49	−6.78	−19.11	4.88	4.16
P	0.01	<0.01	<0.01	<0.01	0.03	0.04

FMC-D, First medical contact to device time; D-B, door to balloon time; FMC-ECG, First medical contact to ECG; ECG-D, ECG to diagnosis.

3.3   Peak Enzyme Value and Time.

The enzyme peak time of the experimental group is earlier than that of control group, and the peak value is lower, and there is statistically difference between two groups (P < 0.05). cTnI peak time [(14.2 ± 3.4) h vs. (16.3 ± 4.6) h, P < 0.05], cTnI peak value [(9.3 ± 2.9) ng/ml vs. (12.3 ± 3.2) ng/ml, P < 0.05].

3.4   EF of Ultrasound.

Values of EF were significantly lower in control group than that in experimental group ($P < 0.05$). EF Value of patients admission within 24 h [(49.3 ± 6.1)% vs. (46.2 ± 7.9)%, $P < 0.05$], EF value after 1 month [(51.3 ± 6.5)% vs. (47.8 ± 6.8)%, $P < 0.05$], EF value after 6 months [(56.7 ± 5.9)% vs. (49.6 ± 6.7)%, $P < 0.05$].

3.5   Heart Failure and Mortality

There is significant difference in in-hospital heart failure between two groups, as well as cardiac mortality after 6 months ($P < 0.05$); but no significant difference in cardiac mortality in hospital or after 1 month ($P > 0.05$). In-hospital heart failure [13 (22.8) vs. 25 (41.0), $P < 0.05$], cardiac mortality after 6 months [2 (3.5) vs. the 9 (14.8), $P < 0.05$], in-hospital mortality [1 (1.8) vs. 3 (4.9), $P > 0.05$], 1 month mortality [1 (1.8) vs. 4 (6.6), $P > 0.05$], 6 month mortality [2 (3.5) vs. 6(9.8), $P > 0.05$].

3.6   Health Economic Parameters

There were significant differences in health economic parameters between two groups ($P < 0.05$); total cost in hospital between two groups [(56711 ± 12083) yuan vs. (65847 ± 14691) yuan, $P < 0.05$], total hospital stay [(6.35 ± 3.68) d vs. the day (8.64 ± 5.19) d, $P < 0.05$].

4   Discussion

"The failure of AMI treatment should be seen as a failure of process and system. The solution lies not only in new drugs or equipment, but also more effective organization methods", said by professor Hu Dayi [7]. Establishment of chest pain center (CPC) has been proved of no effect on improving the FMC-D time of STEMI patient by recent study [8]. After a long time of development, the improvement of hospital emergency system has entered a bottleneck stage. The significant delays for diagnosis of STEMI patients in the first medical consultation mechanism and transport system also have a great impact and effect on the prognosis of patients. This study shows that the establishment of regional cooperation system can significantly shorten the FMC-D time and cTnI peak time, improve heart function of patients, reduce the incidence of heart failure in hospital. Although cardiac mortality of experimental group was lower compared with the control group, but there was no significant difference between the two groups. Revascularization time of the experimental group is shorter than the control group, which reduced the degree of myocardial damage. That is well illustrated by the decreased enzyme peak value, earlier peak time and improved in-hospital cardiac function preservation degree. Relevant study in the whole country has proved the above results [9]. Our study show that Regional Cooperative Rescue System Based on Mobile Internet can significantly shorten the delay of medical system and can maximally improve the prognosis of STEMI patients. This conclusion is also consistent with the current domestic and foreign researches [10, 11]. Regional Cooperative Rescue System, which effectively changes the current STEMI treatment mode and integrates the existing medical resources, better carries out the principle of STEMI treatment "time is heart, heart is life" [12]. In 2012, Mission: Lifeline was started in US, more than 1500 EMS and 450 hospitals in17 main cities were divided into 5 large medical areas. In 2014, Dr. Christopher Granger [11] published the 2 year result of Mission: Lifeline: RCRS shortened the waiting time in emergency room and improve survival rate. By establishment of a standard Regional Cooperative Rescue System in the whole area, the FMC-D time can be significantly improved, and earlier diagnosis and treatment of STEMI can be achieved. And this study shows mobile health and smart health can play a very important role of in the construction of RCRS. Apparently, communication and cooperation between cardiologist and information technologist can lead to more intelligent and efficient treatment for STEMI patient.

References

1. Chen, W.W., Gao, R.L., Liu, L.S., et al.: "Report on cardiovascular diseases in China" Profile. Chin. Circ. J. **07**, 617–622 (2015)
2. Antman, E.M., Hand, M., Armstrong, P.W., et al.: 2007 focused update of the ACC/AHA 2004 guidelines for the management of patients with ST-elevation myocardial infarction: a report of the American College of Cardiology/American Heart Association Task Force on Practice Guidelines. J. Am. Coll. Cardiol. **51**(2), 210–247 (2008)
3. Qin, W.Y.: Establishment of treatment procedure and time management system–the core of Chest pain center construction. In: The Chinese Medical Association Branch of Emergency Medicine 16th National Emergency Medicine Academic Annual Meeting, p. 446. Chinese Medical Association Society of Emergency Medicine, Chinese Medical Association (2014)
4. O'Gara, P.T., Kushner, F.G., Ascheim, D.D., et al.: ACCF/AHA guideline for the management of ST-elevation myocardial infarction: executive summary: a report of the American College of Cardiology Foundation/American Heart Association Task Force on Practice Guidelines. J. Am. Coll. Cardiol. **61**, 485–510 (2013)
5. Chinese Society of Cardiology. The Editorial Board of Chinese Journal of Cardiology: Guidelines on the diagnosis and treatment of acute STEMI. Chin. J. Cardiol. **43**(5), 380–393 (2015)
6. Ge, J.B., Xu, Y.J.: Internal Medicine, p. 224. People's Medical Publishing House, Beijing (2013)
7. Hu, D.Y., Ding, R.J.: Chinese expert consensus about the construction of Chest pain center. Chin. J. Crit. Care Med. **4**(63), 81–393 (2011). (Electronic Edition)
8. Song, L., Yong, Y., Yan, H.B., et al.: Cross-sectional study: referral of patients with STEMI in Beijing. Chin. J. Cardiol. **38**(5), 406–410 (2010)
9. Guo, L.J., Zhao, D.: Analysis of current treatment practice and outcomes for in-patients with ST-segment elevation acute coronary syndrome in 31 provinces of China. J. Peking Univ. (Health Sci.) **43**(3), 440–445 (2011)
10. Wang, X.T., Li, Z.H.: Regionalization network synergy optimizes earlier reperfusion treatment of STEMI. Chin. J. Intervent. Cardiol. **21**(5), 290–296 (2013)
11. Bagai, A., Al-Khalidi, H.R., Sherwood, M.W., et al.: Regional systems of care demonstration project: Mission: Lifeline STEMI Systems Accelerator: design and methodology. Am. Heart J. **167**(1), 15–21, e3 (2014)
12. Hu, D.Y.: Why do we advocate "Green Passage" of Acute Myocardial Infarction. Forum Adv. **8**, 33–34 (2001)

A Robust Algorithm of Encrypted Medical Image Retrieval Based on 3D DFT

Shuangshuang Wang, Jingbing Li$^{(\boxtimes)}$, Chunyan Zhang,
and Zhaohui Wang

College of Information Science and Technology,
Hainan University, Haikou, China
1107132353@qq.com, jingbingli2008@hotmail.com,
13739198205@163.com, william_hig@163.com

Abstract. Cloud computing platform is not a fully trusted third party, which may leak the patient's personal information when we store medical image, so we need to encrypt medical image. Meanwhile, in order to help doctors who can find out historical cases from the medical image database which are similar to the current diagnostic image to make more accurate diagnosis and treatment, this paper proposes an robust algorithm based on 3D DFT for encrypted medical image retrieval. At first, we extract feature vector of 3D encrypted image and establish features vector database. Next, the NC (Normalized Cross Correlation Coefficient) between the feature vector of query medical image and each one in the features vector database is computed automatically. Finally, the corresponding encrypted image with the highest NC value is returned. The results show that this algorithm has strong robustness against common attacks and geometric attacks.

Keywords: 3D medical images · Encrypted medical images retrieval · Feature vector · NC · Robustness

1 Introduction

Doctors draw on both experience and intuition, then using analysis and heuristics to diagnose disease [1]. In clinical medicine, doctors can find out historical cases from the medical image database to make more accurate diagnosis and decide on appropriate treatment. And this is the image retrieval technology. So it is necessary to find an efficient and effective retrieval system. Traditional approach of searching the image was by indexing or simply by browsing. There are some problems with the historical approaches. Thus Content Based Image Retrieval (CBIR) [2–4] emerges at the right moment, which aims at effective searching and browsing a digital image from the large image dataset on the basis of automatically derived image visual features like shape [5], color [6], and texture [7]. Content Based Medical Image Retrieval (CBMIR) also enables to retrieve the medical images from large medical image digital libraries [8]. CBMIR is an automatic retrieve the similar medical images mainly based on the content such as color, composition, shape and texture which is called feature vector. Feature extraction plays an important role in the rapidly and efficient medical image retrieval [9].

© Springer International Publishing AG 2017
C. Xing et al. (Eds.): ICSH 2016, LNCS 10219, pp. 238–250, 2017.
DOI: 10.1007/978-3-319-59858-1_23

As we all know, many hospitals produce a large amount of medical images during diagnosing therapy every day, such as X-rays, CT (Computed Tomography), MRI (Nuclear Magnetic Resource Imaging), ultrasound images and so on, which provide great support to doctors in clinical care. So how to help doctors more rapid and accurate retrieval of the target image, which has become a necessary problem to be solved. More efficient image storage and retrieval services are needed. Cloud computing provides a huge opportunity to access adequate computing and storage resources, which makes it an attractive option for medical image storage [10]. However, Cloud computing platform may leak the patient's personal information, so we need to encrypt medical image. In addition, we hope that the third party cloud computing can complete image retrieval process in the encrypted domain.

How to achieve the image retrieval in the encrypted domain is also a big issue that should be taken into account. When encrypted data are encrypted by general encryption algorithm, we need decrypt at first through the party who has the key when calculate ciphertext data, which will take a high computational cost and communication cost, and reduce the security of information after decrypt. Homomorphical encryption [11] algorithm can solve these problems. Homomorphic encryption, proposed by Rivest et al. [12] in the 70 s of the last century, is a novel encryption algorithm. It has brought a great impact on the world, for example, it is able to blindly compute a search result without revealing its contents [13]. Compared with the general encryption algorithm, homomorphic encryption can implement not only the basic encrypted operations, but also computing over encrypted data and then decrypt rather than decrypting each ciphertext at first. This property is of great significance for the protection of information security.

In this paper, we proposed a robust algorithm of encrypted medical image retrieval based on 3D DFT. It combines 3D DFT transform, Logistic Map and image features extraction in encrypted domain. This algorithm has strong robustness against normal attacks and geometric attacks. It shortens the time of retrieving medical image and improves the efficiency.

2 Fundamental Theory

2.1 3D Discrete Fourier Transform (3D-DFT)

Discrete Fourier Transform is a fundamental transformation in the field of image processing. The size of the medical image is M * N * P, then the three-dimensional Discrete Fourier Transform (3D-DFT) and Inverse Discrete Fourier Transform (3D-IDFT) are defined in formula (1) and (2).

Where f(x, y, z) is the sampling value in the spatial domain, F(u, v, w) is the sampling value in the frequency domain. Medical image can be produced by CT and MRI, which is composed of many layers of the slice, and each slice is a two-dimensional image, the size is M * N, the number of the slice is P.

$$F(u, v, w) = \sum_{x=0}^{M-1}\sum_{y=0}^{N-1}\sum_{z=0}^{P-1} f(x, y, z) \cdot e^{-j2\pi xu/M} e^{-j2\pi yv/N} e^{-j2\pi zw/P} \tag{1}$$

$$u = 0, 1, \cdots, M-1; v = 0, 1, \cdots, N-1; w = 0, 1, \cdots, P-1;$$

$$f(x, y, z) = \frac{1}{MNP}\sum_{u=0}^{M-1}\sum_{v=0}^{N-1}\sum_{w=0}^{P-1} F(u, v, w) \cdot e^{j2\pi xu/M} e^{j2\pi yv/N} e^{j2\pi zw/P} \tag{2}$$

$$x = 0, 1, \cdots, M-1; y = 0, 1, \cdots, N-1; z = 0, 1, \cdots, P-1;$$

2.2   Logistic Map

Logistic map [14, 15] is the most typical and famous, widely used chaotic system, which is a typical one-dimensional chaotic system. For its simple structure and easy to implement, it is widely studied and used, also known as the worm port model. Logistic Map is a nonlinear map given by the following formula:

$$x_{k+1} = \mu x_k(1 - x_k) \tag{3}$$

Where $0 < \mu \le 4$ is the branch parameter, $x_k \in (0, 1)$ is the system variable, the iteration number is K. When $3.5699456\ldots < \mu \le 4$, the system will show a chaotic form. That is to say, if give the initial value x_0, Logistic Map chaotic system will produce a sequence of $\{x_k, k = 1, 2, 3, \ldots\}$, which is very easy to be affected by the initial number x_0. In this paper, $\mu = 4$.

3   The Algorithm Process

3.1   3D Medical Image Encryption

Step1: At first, the original 3D medical image is processed using 3D-DFT (3D Discrete Fourier Transform), obtaining complex number coefficient matrix FD(i, j, k);

$$FD(i, j, k) = DFT3(F(i, j, k)) \tag{4}$$

Step2: Set the initial value x_0, a one-dimensional chaotic sequence bl(j) is generated by Logistic Map chaotic system;

Step3: Define a threshold symbol function Sign(i), then turn bl(j) into binary chaotic sequence only contains 1 and −1 and construct a binary matrix S(i, j, k) whose size is same as F(i, j, k), $1 \le i \le M, 1 \le j \le N, 1 \le k \le P$

$$Sign(bl(j)) = \begin{cases} 1 & bl(j) > 0.5 \\ -1 & bl(j) \le 0.5 \end{cases} \tag{5}$$

Step4: Then do a dot products between the complex number coefficient matrix FD (i, j, k) and binary matrix S(i, j, k), get a matrix L(i, j, k);

$$L(i,j,k) = FD(i,j,k). * S(i,j,k) \tag{6}$$

Step5: Use 3D-IDFT (3D Inverse Discrete Fourier Transform) for L(i, j, k), then obtain the encrypted medical image E(i, j, k);

$$E(i,j,k) = IDFT3(L(i,j,k)) \tag{7}$$

3.2 Extract the Feature Vector of 3D Encrypted Medical Image

Firstly, the encrypted 3D medical image E(i, j, k) is computed using 3D-DFT, getting complex number coefficient matrix ED(i, j, k); Then the first m × n × p complex number matrix coefficients are selected, we can regard one complex number as the real part and the imaginary part two numbers, we will get 2 × m × n × p numbers, then place them in a sequence, define a threshold symbol function Sign(j), obtain the feature vector, which is consists of 0, 1. In this case, we chose m = n = 2, p = 1, then we get a sequence of numbers '10110110' which is the feature vector of the original encrypted 3D medical image. After observing the Table 1, we can find that under common attacks and geometric attacks, the NC between feature vector after attacks and the original one is 1.0. When the 3D medical image is under proper common attacks, this vector

Table 1. Part of coefficients of encrypted images and values after different attacks

	Image manipula-tion	PSNR (dB)	ED(1,1,1)	ED(1,2,1)	ED(2,1,1)	ED(2,2,1)	symbolic sequence	NC
Common attack	Original encrypted image		3.47+0.00i	0.79+0.07i	-0.15+0.05i	0.03-0.01i	10110110	1.0
	Gaussian noise (1%)	20.24	3.49+0.00i	0.78+0.06i	-0.15+0.05i	0.03-0.01i	10110110	1.0
	JPEG compression (4%)	22.46	3.46+0.00i	0.80+0.06i	-0.15+0.05i	0.04-0.01i	10110110	1.0
	Median filtering [5x5]	21.05	3.31+0.00i	0.72+0.07i	-0.21+0.04i	0.02-0.01i	10110110	1.0
Geometric attack	Anticlockwise rotation(5°)	17.15	3.30+0.00i	0.63+0.05i	-0.21+0.02i	0.06-0.04i	10110110	1.0
	Scaling(2)		13.88+0.00i	3.18+0.22i	-0.59+0.20i	0.14-0.04i	10110110	1.0
	Scaling(0.5)		0.87+0.00i	0.20+0.02i	-0.04+0.01i	0.01-0.002i	10110110	1.0
	Down shift(5%)	16.74	3.32+0.00i	0.77+0.07i	-0.27+0.11i	0.004-0.02i	10110110	1.0
	Left shift(5%)	14.93	3.19+0.00i	0.45+0.27i	-0.13+0.03i	0.06-0.01i	10110110	1.0
	Cropping(10%,Z direction)		3.08+0.00i	0.71+0.06i	-0.14+0.04i	0.02-0.004i	10110110	1.0

The unit of the coefficients processed by 3D DFT is 1.0e+07

remains almost unchanged. For geometric attacks, part of coefficient value has great change, but it is easy to notice that its symbol is not changed.

In order to further prove that the feature vector extracted by the above method is an important feature of the 3D encrypted medical image. We also did experiments among different 3D images (shown as Fig. 1(a)-(f)) and their encrypted images (shown as Fig. 2(a)-(f)). By observing Table 2, firstly, the correlation coefficient between the encrypted data itself is the largest, which is 1.00; Secondly, the correlation coefficient between the similar images is larger for 0.35, and the shape of the images before encryption which correspond to the two images is similar, both which are liver volume data; Thirdly, the correlation coefficient between the feature vectors of other encrypted data is small, for their images before encryption is not similar, which is consistent with what our human eyes observe. So we can come to the conclusion that the feature vector

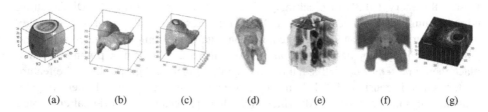

(a)   (b)   (c)   (d)   (e)   (f)   (g)

Fig. 1. Different 3D medical images: (a) head; (b) liver1; (c) liver2; (d) teeth; (e) engine; (f) teddy bear; (g) echo

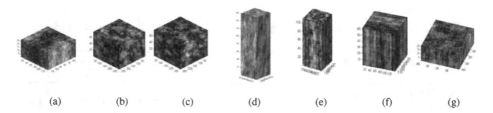

(a)   (b)   (c)   (d)   (e)   (f)   (g)

Fig. 2. Different 3D encrypted medical images: (a) head; (b) liver1; (c) liver2; (d) teeth; (e) engine; (f) teddy bear; (g) echo

Table 2. NC between feature vector of different 3D encrypted medical images

	Va	Vb	Vc	Vd	Ve	Vf	Vg
Va	1.00	0.26	0.03	0.05	0.03	−0.12	0.10
Vb	0.26	1.00	0.35	0.07	0.16	−0.13	−0.29
Vc	0.03	0.35	1.00	−0.09	0.06	0.16	0.06
Vd	0.05	0.07	−0.09	1.00	0.03	−0.19	−0.09
Ve	0.03	0.16	0.06	0.03	1.00	0.03	0.00
Vf	−0.12	−0.13	0.16	−0.19	0.03	1.00	0.03
Vg	0.10	−0.29	0.06	−0.09	0.00	0.03	1.00

computed by the algorithm in this paper can reflect the main feature of the 3D encrypted medical image.

3.3   Establish Feature Vector Database of 3D Encrypted Medical Images

Step1: Obtain feature vectors EV(j) of 3D encrypted medical images
   The 3D encrypted medical images in the image database E = {E1, E2,...,EN} are processed using 3D DFT separately and each DFT complex number coefficient matrix ED(i, j, k) is got; the first $4 \times 4 \times 2$ complex number coefficients are selected, obtaining complex number matrix ED'(i, j, k), and then we regard one complex number as the real part and the imaginary part two numbers, thus, $2 \times 4 \times 4 \times 2$ numbers are got; then place them in a sequence, getting a one dimensional real matrix ED''(j), define a threshold symbol function Sign(j), obtaining the feature vector EV(j) of 3D encrypted medical image to be retrieval, which is consists of 0, 1.
   Step2: Store the feature vector EV(j) of the 3D encrypted medical images in the feature vector database EV = {EV1, EV2,..., EVN}.

$$ED(i,j,k) = DFT3(E(i,j,k)) \tag{8}$$

$$Sign(ED''(j)) = \begin{cases} 1 & ED''(j) > 0 \\ 0 & ED''(j) \leq 0 \end{cases} \tag{9}$$

3.4   The Automatic Retrieval of 3D Encrypted Medical Images

The model of 3D encrypted medical images retrieval is shown in the Fig. 3.
   Step 1. Encrypt 3D medical image $F'(i,j,k)$ to acquire the 3D encrypted medical image $E'(i,j,k)$;
   Step 2. Obtain the feature vector $EV'(j)$;
   Step 3. Compute NC between $EV'(j)$ and EV(j);
   The Normalized Cross-correlation (NC) is used to compute the similarity between two images. Each NC between $EV'(j)$ and EV(j) in the feature vector database is computed. The value of NC is larger, the retrieved images and the original images are more similar. The formula of NC is as follows:

$$NC = \frac{\sum_j w(j)w'(j)}{\sum_j w(j)w(j)} \tag{10}$$

Step 4. Return the 3D encrypted medical image according to the highest NC.

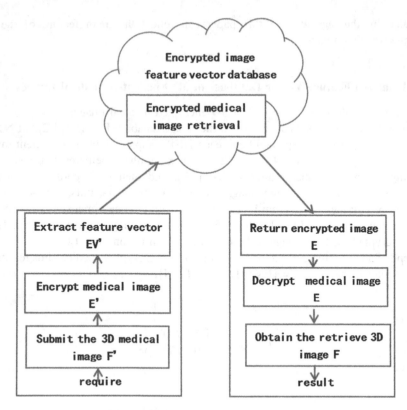

Fig. 3. The 3D encrypted medical images retrieval model

4 The Experimental Results

In this paper, the simulation platform is Matlab2014a, we choose the MRI data which belongs to MTLAB to do the experiment, and we use 1000 groups of independent binary pseudo-random sequences, which include +1 and 0, the length of every group is 64bits. We put the feature vector of the target medical image in the 500th group choosing from the 1000 groups data. The purpose of the experiment is to test and validate whether the target medical image can be retrieved by the algorithm when the image to be retrieved is under attacks. The original medical image and original encrypted medical image can be expressed as F(i, j, k) and E(i, j, k) showing in the Fig. 4(a) and (b), in which $1 \leq i, j \leq 128, 1 \leq k \leq 27$. 3D DFT coefficient matrix of original encrypted image is ED(I, j, k), from which the feature vector of the encrypted image can be obtained. Then, by computing NC value we can retrieve the similar images.

PSNR (Peak Signal to Noise Ratio) is the most widely used to objectively evaluate image quality. In this paper, we use PSNR to objectively evaluate quality of the image to be retrieved after attacks, which is defined as:

$$PSNR = 10 \lg \left[\frac{MN \max_{i,j}(\mathrm{I}(i,j))^2}{\sum_i \sum_j (\mathrm{I}(i,j) - \mathrm{I}'(i,j))^2} \right] \tag{11}$$

In the experiment, when we put the original encrypted 3D medical image into feature vector detector, then the output is shown in the Fig. 4(c), from which we can find that NC reach the peak in the 500th group, the corresponding image is shown in the Fig. 4(d).

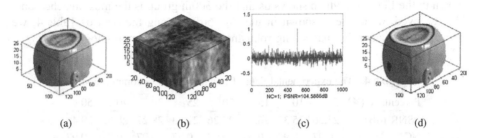

(a)   (b)   (c)   (d)

Fig. 4. The original encrypted medical image and the result of retrieving (a) the original encrypted slice image; (b) the corresponding 3D encrypted images; (c) detector response; (d) the retrieved image.

4.1 Common Attacks

(1) Interference of Gaussian Noise

We add Gaussian noise to the original encrypted image by using the function of imnoise(). Figure 5(a) is an original image when Gaussian noise intensity is 1%, which has a little vague. And the corresponding encrypted image is shown in the Fig. 5(b). When we put it into detector, the response is shown in the Fig. 5(c), we can see that the maximum NC value of the detector appears in the 500th groups, the retrieved image is shown in the Fig. 5(d). From Table 3, when Gaussian noise intensity is 20%, NC = 0.82, the image also can be retrieved easily. That is to say, this algorithm has strong anti-Gaussian noise ability.

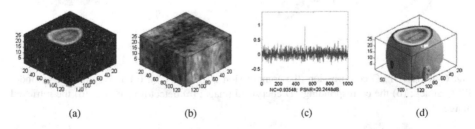

(a)   (b)   (c)   (d)

Fig. 5. Under Gaussian noise (the noise intensity is 1%): (a) an original image under Gaussian noise; (b) the corresponding 3D encrypted image; (c) detector response; (d) the retrieved image.

Table 3. The experimental data of image anti-Gaussian noise

Noise intensity (%)	1	3	5	8	10	15	20
PSNR (dB)	20.23	15.84	13.96	12.32	11.61	10.41	9.66
NC	0.97	0.94	0.94	0.94	0.87	0.91	0.82

(2) JPEG compression attacks

Figure 6(a) is an original image under JPEG attack (the compression quality is 4%), from which we can see obvious difference with clear blocking effects, the corresponding 3D encrypted image is shown in the Fig. 6(b). The response of detector is shown in the Fig. 6(c), which shows us that the 500th group is the most matched one. The retrieved 3D image is shown in the Fig. 6(d). Seeing the data of Table 4, we know that this algorithm has strong robustness anti-JPEG compression attacks.

Table 4. The experimental data of image anti-JPEG compression

Percentage (%)	5	10	15	20	25	30	40	50
PSNR (dB)	23.20	25.37	26.52	27.26	27.83	28.27	28.93	29.48
NC	0.97	0.97	0.94	0.97	0.97	0.97	0.97	0.97

(3) Median filtering attacks

In the experiment, we test the filter impact on the encrypted medical image by changing the size of median filters and filtering number of repeats, these data are shown in Table 5. The original image under median filtering [5 × 5] (10 times) is shown in Fig. 7(a), from which we can find that the image is very vague. The 3D encrypted image under attack is shown in Fig. 7(b). From Fig. 7(c) we know that the detector can retrieve the 500th feature vector value obviously, the retrieved 3D image is shown in the Fig. 7(d), which shows this algorithm has strong robustness against median filtering attacks.

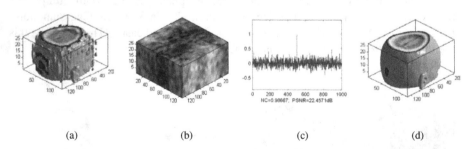

(a)   (b)   (c)   (d)

Fig. 6. Under JPEG compression (the compression quality is 4%): (a) an original image under JPEG attack; (b) the corresponding 3D encrypted image; (c) detector response; (d) the retrieved image.

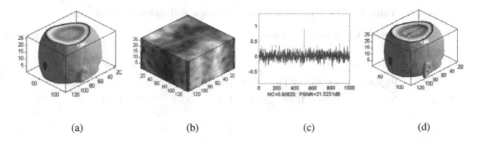

(a)   (b)   (c)   (d)

Fig. 7. Under Median filtering (Median filtering [5 × 5] repeating 10 times): (a) an original image under Median filtering; (b) the corresponding 3D encrypted image; (c) detector response; (d) the retrieved image.

Table 5. The experimental data of image anti-Median filtering

	Median filtering [3 x 3]			Median filtering [5 x 5]			Median filtering [7 x 7]		
Repeating times	1	2	10	1	2	10	1	2	10
PSNR(dB)	27.40	26.56	24.95	24.57	23.74	21.52	22.98	22.32	20.13
NC	1.00	1.00	1.00	1.00	0.94	0.91	0.94	0.94	0.86

4.2   Geometrical Attacks

(1) Rotation attacks

When the original image is under Rotation (anticlockwise 5°), which is shown in the Fig. 8(a). The 3D encrypted image under attack is shown in Fig. 8(b), PSNR = 17.15 dB. When we put it into the detector, the biggest output in the 500th feature vector value is shown in the Fig. 8(c). The retrieved 3D image is shown in the Fig. 8 (d). From the Table 6, when the image is rotated 10°(clockwise), NC = 0.59, the image also can be retrieved. So we can draw such a conclusion that this algorithm has good anti-Rotation attacks ability.

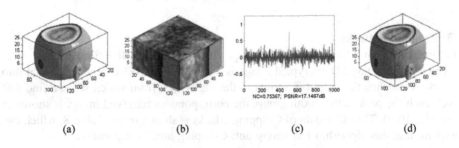

(a)   (b)   (c)   (d)

Fig. 8. Under Rotation (anticlockwise 5°): (a) an original image under rotation; (b) the corresponding 3D encrypted image; (c) detector response; (d) the retrieved image.

Table 6. The experimental data of image anti-Rotation attacks

Rotation	Clockwise rotation				Anticlockwise rotation		
Degree (°)	−10°	−5°	−1°	0°	1°	5°	10°
PSNR(dB)	15.26	17.11	23.89	104.59	23.90	17.15	15.28
NC	0.59	0.73	0.91	1.00	0.91	0.76	0.51

(2) Scaling attacks

The scaling factor is used as a parameter in the scaling attacks experiment. Figure 9(a) shows an original image with a scale factor of 0.5. The encrypted image under attack is shown in Fig. 9(b). From Fig. 9(c) we know that the detector can retrieve the 500th feature vector value easily. The retrieved image is shown in the Fig. 9(d). Table 7 can prove that algorithm our proposed has strong robustness against scaling attacks.

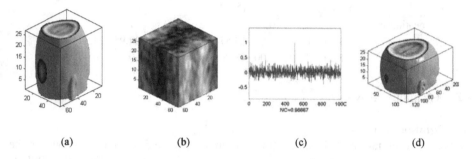

(a)	(b)	(c)	(d)

Fig. 9. Under scaling(0.5): (a) an original image under scaling; (b) the corresponding 3D encrypted image; (c) detector response; (d) the retrieved image.

Table 7. The experimental data of image anti-Scaling attacks

Scaling	0.2	0.5	0.8	1.00	1.2	1.5	2.0	4.0
NC	0.75	0.97	0.97	1.00	1.00	1.00	1.00	1.00

(3) Cropping attacks

Figure 10(a) shows that the original image cropping from Z direction, 10%
. The corresponding 3D encrypted image is shown in Fig. 10(b). When we put it into the detector, then the output is shown in the Fig. 10(c), from which we can find that NC reach the peak in the 500th group, the corresponding retrieved image is shown in the Fig. 10(d). The other data of Cropping attacks is shown in the Table 8, which can explain that this algorithm has strong anti-Cropping attacks capability.

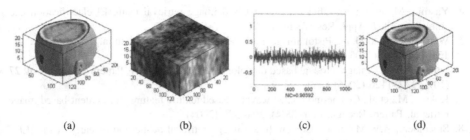

(a)   (b)   (c)   (d)

Fig. 10. Under cropping attack (z 10%): (a) an original image under cropping; (b) the corresponding 3D encrypted image; (c) detector response; (d) the retrieved image.

Table 8. The experimental data of image anti-Cropping attacks

	Ratio(%)	2	4	6	8	10	12	14	16	18	20
Z	NC	0.97	0.97	0.87	0.87	0.91	0.91	0.84	0.84	0.81	0.81
Y	NC	0.81	0.79	0.78	0.70	0.63	0.47	0.47	0.44	0.37	0.44
X	NC	0.91	0.84	0.75	0.75	0.79	0.78	0.62	0.59	0.59	0.56

5 Conclusions

This paper proposes a robust algorithm of 3D encrypted medical image retrieval, which combines 3D DFT transform, Logistic Map and image features extraction in encrypted domain. The experimental results show that this algorithm has ideal robustness against Gaussian noise, JPEG compression, Median filtering, Rotation, Scaling, Cropping attacks. Meanwhile, this algorithm also protects patient's information in cipher domain. Moreover, it has quicker retrieval speed and good practicability.

Acknowledgments. This work is supported by the National Natural Science Foundation of China (No: 61263033), and by the International Science and Technology Cooperation Project of Hainan (No: KJHZ2015-04, KJHZ2015-23) and the Institutions of Higher Learning Scientific Research Special Project of Hainan Province (NO: Hnkyzx2014-2).

References

1. Yang, L., et al.: A boosting framework for visuality-preserving distance metric learning and its application to medical image retrieval. IEEE Trans. Pattern Anal. Mach. Intell. **32**(1), 30–44 (2010)
2. Rao, L.K., et al.: Content based medical image retrieval using local co-occurrence patterns. In: IEEE International Conference on Applied and Theoretical Computing and Communication Technology (iCATccT), pp. 743–748 (2015)
3. Jyothi, B., et al.: An effective multiple visual features for content based medical image retrieval. In: 9th International Conference on Intelligent Systems and Control (ISCO), pp. 1–5. IEEE (2015)

4. Yasmin, M., et al.: An efficient content based image retrieval using EI classification and color features. J. Appl. Res. Technol. **12**(5), 877–885 (2014)

5. Wen, C.Y., Yao, J.Y.: Pistol image retrieval by shape representation. Forensic Sci. Int. **155**(1), 35–50 (2005)

6. Sun, J.D., et al.: Image retrieval based on color distribution entropy. Pattern Recogn. Lett. **27** (10), 1122–1126 (2006)

7. Kokare, M., et al.: Cosine-modulated wavelet based texture features for content-based image retrieval. Pattern Recogn. Lett. **25**(4), 391–398 (2004)

8. Smeulders, A.W.M., et al.: Content-based image retrieval at the end of early years. IEEE Trans. Pattern Anal. Mach. Intell. **22**(12), 1349–1380 (2000)

9. Murthy, V.S., et al.: content based image retrieval using hierarchical and kmeans clustering techniques. Int. J. Eng. Sci. Technol. **2**(3), 209–212 (2010)

10. Xia, Z.H., et al.: A privacy-preserving and copy-deterrence content-based image retrieval scheme in cloud computing. IEEE Trans. Inf. Forensics Secur. **PP**(99), 1 (2016)

11. Bellafqira, R., et al.: Content-based image retrieval in homomorphic encryption domain. In: 37th Annual International Conference of the IEEE Engineering in Medicine and Biology Society (EMBC), pp. 2944–2947 (2015)

12. Rivest, R., et al.: On data banks and privacy homomorphisms. In: Foundations of Secure Computation, pp. 169–180 (1978)

13. Palamakumbura, S., Usefi, H.: Database query privacy using homomorphic encryptions. In: IEEE 14th Canadian Workshop on Information Theory (CWIT), pp. 71–74 (2015)

14. Sun, Y., Wang, G.Y.: An image encryption scheme based on modified logistic map. In: Fourth International Workshop on Chaos-Fractals Theories and Applications (IWCFTA), pp. 179–182 (2011)

15. Zhang, X.F., Fan, J.L.: Extended logistic chaotic sequence and its performance analysis. Tsinghua Sci. Technol. **12**(S1), 156–161 (2007)

Erratum to: Classification of Cataract Fundus Image Based on Retinal Vascular Information

Yanyan Dong[1], Qing Wang[2], Qinyan Zhang[1], and Jijiang Yang[2(✉)]

[1] Automation School, Beijing University of Post and Telecommunications, Beijing, China
dyy0506@bupt.edu.cn, zh_qinyan@163.com
[2] Research Institute of Information Technology, Tsinghua University, Beijing 100084, China
qing.wang@tsinghua.edu.cn, yangjijiang@tsingha.edu.cn

Erratum to:
Chapter "Classification of Cataract Fundus Image Based on Retinal Vascular Information" in:
C. Xing et al. (Eds.): Smart Health, LNCS 10219,
https://doi.org/10.1007/978-3-319-59858-1_16

The initially published version of authors' affiliations was incorrect.

The updated online version of this chapter can be found at
https://doi.org/10.1007/978-3-319-59858-1_16

© Springer International Publishing AG 2017
C. Xing et al. (Eds.): ICSH 2016, LNCS 10219, p. E1, 2017.
https://doi.org/10.1007/978-3-319-59858-1_24

Author Index

Printed in the United States
By Bookmasters